Introduction to Oriental Medicine
through Charts and Graphs
The Missing Charts Manual

ISBN 0-9747531-0-6

Printed in the United States by:
OREGON LITHOPRINT Inc.

Distributed by:
Zdenek Zumr LAc.
1024 SW Troy St.
Portland, OR 97219
zzumr@aol.com

This book is an introduction to Oriental Medicine and is not
intended for the diagnosis and/or treatment of illness. It is
not to replace the skills of a trained health care provider.

Permission to reprint the Zang/Fu charts from:
John McDonald and Joel Penner from:
ZANG FU SYNDROMES: DIFFERENTIAL DIAGNOSIS AND
TREATMENT, published by Lone Wolf Press, 1994

For my dad, the Engineer

Outline i
About the Author iv
Layout v
Introduction vi
        Chinese versus Oriental Medicine vi
Chinsese Medicine 1
   History, 4000 years in 15 minutes 1
     Origin 1
     The Three Pillars 1
       At Home 1
       The Masters 1
       Institutions 1
   Recent History 2
     Cultural Revolution 2
     Migration to the West 2
   Foundations 3
                  Graphic: Foundations of TCM 3
     Tao, before the Division 4
     Yin/Yang, First Division 5
                  Graphic: Yin Yang Complimentary Pairs 5
                  Graphic: Yin/Yang Relationships and Expressions 6
       Pathologies 6
     Three Treasures 7
                  Graphic: Three Treasures 7
       Shen 7
       Jing 8
                  Graphic: Jing Store 8
                  Graphic: Jing Balance 9
       Qi 10
                  Graphic: Qi v/s Energy 10
       What is "Qi" 11
       Generation 12
                  Graphic: Generation of Qi 12
       Function 13
                  Graphic: Five Functions of Qi 13
     Other Substances Involved 14
       Xue 14
               Graphic: Xue 14
       Yin/Ye 15
     5 Elements, Second Division 17
                  Graphic: Five Elements 17
       Interactions 19
                  Graphic: Five Element Interactions (1) 19
                  Graphic: Five Element Interactions (2) 20
                  Graphic: Possible Five Element Arrangements 21
                  Graphic: Element Date 22
       Feng Shui. 23
                  Graphic: Geomancy Compass 21
     12 Meridians, Third Division 25
                  Graphic: Meridian Flow 25
                  Graphic: Spiral Clock 26
                  Graphic: 24 Hour Progression 27
       Zang / Fu 28

Graphic: Zang / Fu 28
Graphic: Physical / Conceptual aspects of TCM 29
Meridians 31
Graphic: Lung Meridian 32
Graphic: Zang / Fu Syndromes: Lung 33
Graphic: Large Intestine Meridian 34
Graphic: Zang / Fu Syndromes: Large Intestine 35
Graphic: Stomach Meridian 36
Graphic: Zang / Fu Syndromes: Stomach 37
Graphic: Spleen Meridian 38
Graphic: Zang / Fu Syndromes: Spleen 39
Graphic: Heart Meridian 40
Graphic: Zang / Fu Syndromes: Heart 41
Graphic: Small Intestine Meridian 42
Graphic: Zang / Fu Syndromes: Small Intestine 43
Graphic: Urinary Bladder Meridian 44
Graphic: Zang / Fu Syndromes: Urinary Bladder 45
Graphic: Kidney Meridian 46
Graphic: Zang / Fu Syndromes: Kidney 47
Graphic: Pericardium Meridian................................. 48
Graphic: San Jiao Meridian 49
Graphic: Gall Bladder Meridian 50
Graphic: Zang / Fu Syndromes: Gall Bladder 51
Graphic: Liver Meridian 52
Graphic: Zang / Fu Syndromes: Liver 53
Eight Extras... 54
Graphic: Ren Meridian 55
Graphic: Du Meridian 56
Pathogenesis 58
Six External Pathogens 58
Internal Pathologies 58
Graphic: Seven Emotions 58
Pathologies of Qi 59
Other Factors 60
Diet 60
Lifestyle 60
Trauma 60
Wrong Treatment 61
Diagnosis 61
Graphic: Eight Differentiations 63
Treatment Modalities 63
Acupuncture 63
Moxa 64
Manual Techniques 64
Shiatsu 65
JinShinDo 65
Tui-Na 65
An-ma 65
Cupping 65
GuaSha 67
Herbs 67
Graphic: Pure, Herbal, Natural, = Healthy? 68
Diet 68

Graphic: Western Food Pyramid 69
Graphic: TCM Food Pyramid 70
Graphic: Vegetarian Food Pyramid 71
Spiritual Practices 72
Lifestyle 73
Graphic: Healing Pyramid 74
Valuable point selections for the massage therapist 75
Ayurvedic medicine 77
The Five Elements 78
Graphic: Ayurvedic Five Elements 78
Doshas 79
Graphic: Doshas 79
Vata 80
Pita 81
Kapha 81
Graphic: 24 Hour Doshas 81
Archetypes/Constitutions 82
Graphic: Archetypes 82
Single 83
Dual 83
Tripple 83
Pathogenesis 84
Graphic: Pathogenesis 84
Maintaining Agni 85
Treatment Approach 86
Sattvic life style 86
Ayurvedic Remedies 86
Auras, Chakras 89
Auras 90
Graphic: Radiating Auras 90
Graphic: Distinct Layers Auras 91
Aura Layers 92
Chakras 93
Chakra #1, Base 94
Chakra #2, Sacral 94
Chakra #3, Solar Plexus 95
Chakra #4, Heart 95
Graphic: Heart Chakra Pivot 96
Chakra #5, Throat 97
Chakra #6, Third Eye 97
Chakra #7, Crown 98
Chakra Summary Table 99
Graphic: The Chakras 100
Addendum .... A
TCM Booklist .... A
Booklist for Ayurveda .... B
TCM Schools C
Quiz 1 .... D
Quiz 2 .... F
Quiz 3 .... H
Quiz 4 .... J

Zdenek Zumr L.Ac.

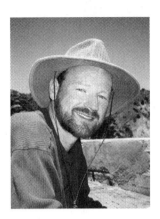

Zdenek Zumr was born in Czechoslovakia, but left with his family after the spring revolution of '68. After a few years in Morocco they moved to Switzerland and acquired citizenship. Educated in electronics engineering his work sent him around the globe.

During one such journey he encountered Shiatsu massage. Intrigued he spent a year learning about Shiatsu and Chinese medicine. In 1993 he changed careers to pursue full time study of Traditional Chinese Medicine and graduated from Yo San University with a Master Degree in Traditional Chinese Medicine and Acupuncture in 1997.

Since September 1998, Zdenek has lived in Portland Oregon, where he practices Chinese medicine at the Pearl Clinic, a multidisciplinary clinic and pharmacy that includes western, eastern and naturopathic doctors as well as psychologists, bodyworkers and clinical estheticians.

For more information about the practice look up: **www.pearlclinic.com** or **www.thepearlpharmacy.com**

Besides his practice and teaching he also publishes instructional materials for Oriental Medicine schools.

A collection of flow charts and graphics was published in the book: ZANG FU SYNDROMES: DIFFERENTIAL DIAGNOSIS AND TREATMENT
by John McDonald and Joel Penner
published by Lone Wolf Press, P.O. 2635 Toluca Lake, CA 91610
ISBN: 0-9650529-0-7
www.amaricandragon.com

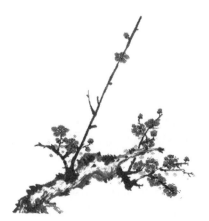

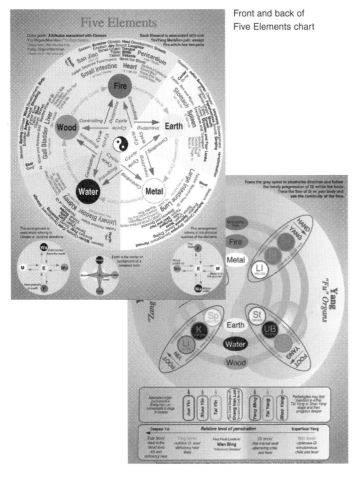

Front and back of
Five Elements chart

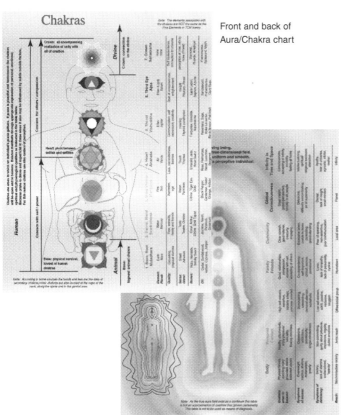

Front and back of
Aura/Chakra chart

Purpose

The purpose of this workbook is to provide students an introduction to the basic tenets of Oriental medicine with emphasis on Traditional Chinese Medicine (TCM), its terminology and ways to organize information. It also contains key elements of Ayurvedic medicine as well as a brief description of the Chakra/Aura system. It is meant to provide students with enough information to pass the "Oriental Medicine" portion of the Washington and Oregon massage board exams and to broaden their perspectives on the subject of medicine and health care.

Invitation

Oriental Medicine is an extremely broad subject and there are many schools of thought. This workbook concentrates on concepts that are universally accepted by most schools. For the purpose of brevity generalizations are employed. References to published books are provided for students that intend to broaden their understanding of the subject. As this is work in progress I invite you, my students and fellow instructors, to provide feedback, references and, if need be, corrections to this workbook. Contact **zzumr@aol.com**.

Organization

First, a brief overview is provided to clarify the term "Asian/Oriental Medicine", then a structure is laid out to provide a foundation for information and personal studies. Prose is kept brief and all overheads are referenced in the table of contents for quick review. The addendums contain extra information and a book list provides suggestions for additional readings. Wide margins allow for personal notes and doodles. Quizzes at the end provide feedback on how you're doing.

Charts

The graphics in this workbook are available in the form of an Instructor Graphic Set containing 61 overhead foils, or as a Power Point presentation on CD-Rom.

- Introduction to Oriental Medicine, Charts and Graphs Overhead Set, ISBN: 0-9747531-1-4
- Introduction to Oriental Medicine, Charts and Graphs on CD-ROM, ISBN: 0-9747531-2-2

Two full color, laminated student charts to accompany instruction: Five Elements and Chakra/Aura are available in 8½ x 11 format.
- Five Elements laminated chart, ISBN: 0-9747531-3-0
- Aura/Chakra Laminated chart, ISBN: 0-9747531-4-9

To order contact the author.

This workbook is not meant to be a manual on how to diagnose or treat disorders.

Oriental Medicine

Chinese versus Oriental Medicine

Oriental Medicine encompasses many types of medical practices that arose and are practiced in Asia. Some types of medicine are recognized by country of origin, i.e. Tibetan or Chinese, by treatment method, i.e. acupuncture, cupping, TuiNa, by the philosophy that governs its principles, Ayurvedic, Tantric, Zen, or by family lineage that documented or developed its own form of medicine.

For the purpose of this course we focus on two distinct philosophies, that of Traditional Chinese Medicine (TCM) and Ayurvedic medicine. Either medicine allows the practitioner to diagnose disorders, select a treatment method, administer and modify treatments, and make predictions as to the outcome.

TCM forms the foundation for many medicines in Southeast Asia and is well documented. On that foundation many national styles evolved, including Korean, Japanese medicine.

Treatment methods of TCM include acupuncture which has received much attention and recognition in the West, but also includes herbs, exercises (Tai Qi, Qi Gong and martial arts), hands-on practices such as Shiatsu, An-ma, Jin Shin Do, Tui Na, and others, as well as life style counseling.

Ayurvedic medicine is widely practiced on the Indian sub-continent and is based on its own distinct philosophy. It also includes herbs, exercises and emotional/spiritual counseling.

"The value of the Chinese theories is in aiding the organization of observation, discerning patterns, capturing interconnectedness and qualities of being. Can one prove a poetic image? It can be shared. It can be used. One can decide if it's worth listening to. ..."

Ted J. Kaptchuk

Chinese Medicine
History 4000 years in 15 minutes

Origin

The written history of Traditional Chinese Medicine (TCM) dates back about 4000 years. In this time span, myths and facts merge and the Chinese are not concerned with sorting one from the other.

Thousands of years ago Huang Di "The Yellow Emperor" commissioned a book on then current medical knowledge. This book was called Nei Jing. It contained only a few acupuncture points but many herbs. Over centuries, critiques of Nei Jing were written and after a few centuries, a new standard text was compiled that included a consensus of the critiques. That new text would again invite critiques and a new text would be written. This process repeated itself many times over until this day. In TCM, information is rarely discarded as wrong, but rather information is specified to be correct only under certain circumstances.

The Three Pillars

The sources of Chinese medical information can be divided into three categories. These are the three pillars on which TCM stands: Home, The Masters, and Institutions.

Home

Traditional family remedies have always been utilized and passed down through generations. These remedies include dietary advise, such as chicken soup for colds, herbs, like ginger for nausea, or manual techniques such as massage or salt rubs. Typically these remedies utilize readily available, local supplies for pathological conditions that arise in a particular region. These remedies kept the family healthy through seasonal and life changes.

The Masters

For more complex problems, consults with healers were needed. These were persons that had a broader knowledge of interactions and use of rare herbs for pathological conditions. (Shamans, Midwifes, spiritual healers) This knowledge was taught only to few students with a lifetime commitment. This was a slow, non-methodical approach that maintained secret knowledge in lineages or family clans.

Institutions

TCM Schools originated with monasteries where martial arts developed as a form of self defense. Prevention and care of communicable disease and sanitation became an issue in the monasteries as many people started living in close quarters. With fighting techniques the monks also learned and taught ways to heal wounds sustained in sparring and battle. This was the first time medicine was documented and taught systematically. But it still took many years to learn and only few actually ventured out to help common people. These schools were still secretive and rare. Different schools of thought and style originated depending on environment, climate and politics and each style came with its respective remedies.

- Crane style martial arts was developed where water was present
- Monkey style was developed in jungles
- Ground fighting was developed on slippery slopes

These remedies would be picked up by "Barefoot Doctors" who traveled from town to town. They were often monks that opted out of monastic life or students in search of a master or devotees that took it upon themselves to learn and practice medicine with common people.

With these doctors, medical knowledge was disseminated beyond local boundaries and brought to the attention of scribes who then collected the knowledge to write reference books.

Recent History

The system has survived the warring states period, about 300 years of civil war, colonialism, influx of foreigners in the 17th through 20th century, and World War II.

Cultural Revolution

However Chinese medicine was nearly wiped out by communists during the Cultural Revolution when the "new man" was proclaimed to be free of superstition, religion and tradition. Monasteries were destroyed; millions of people were resettled and forced into labor. Resettled people, unaccustomed to local and climatic conditions and ignorant of traditional local cures, succumbed to infectious disease.

Tai Qi and traditional medicine were forbidden and only few western-trained doctors were allowed to practice. Western-trained doctors had neither the manpower nor resources to take care of the masses. As an emergency measure, the communist government sought out old masters and brought them together to develop a curriculum of traditional Chinese medicine that could be taught quickly to thousands of students.

This was the first teachable, public system of Chinese medicine. However it contains only the most basic elements that the old masters could agree on. The system also excluded any reference to spiritual, religious, and even mental aspects that conflicted with communist dogma.

Migration to the West

Chinese Medicine migrated with Chinese laborers to the US in the 19th century. However, because of racial discrimination and persecution, it remained accessible only to Chinese people that knew of its benefits.

Other countries, such as France and Germany, learned about Chinese medicine through their involvement in Indochina. The knowledge was brought back to Europe for further study. However, TCM remained trapped in academic circles and was never introduced to the public as a form of medicine.

Chinese Medicine entered public awareness in the western hemisphere in the 1970's when a reporter for the New York Times had to undergo an emergency appendectomy while on assignment in China. The main method of pain control was through acupuncture and he remained conscious throughout the procedure.

Today the United States has the strongest following of Chinese Medicine outside of China and many old masters and families have come to this country to engage in a process of reintegrating lost values into Chinese Medicine. Many western medical schools now have introductions to Chinese medicine in the curriculum and acupuncture schools conduct clinical research at hospitals.

Although Chinese medicine can be taught in four years it still takes a lifetime commitment to learn.

Foundations

Graphic: Foundations of TCM

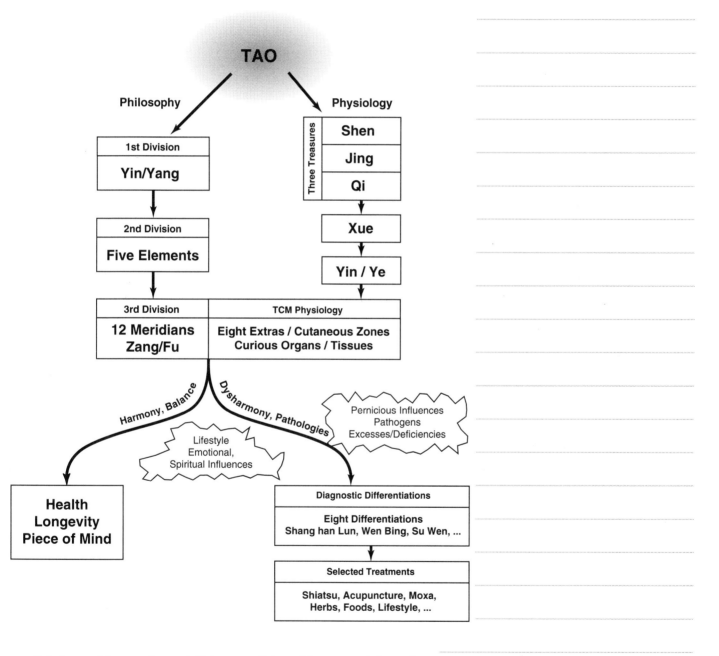

It is impossible to understand Chinese medicine without some information on Chinese philosophy. The same way of thinking that governs all aspects of life, society, art, etc., in China, also governs medicine. The borders between what is medical theory and practice and what is not aren't clearly delineated.

Concepts of **Qi** and **Yin/Yang** form the foundation in all schools of Chinese Medicine, but medicine is only one narrow application of these concepts. The same Qi, Yin and Yang are also used in the context of **Feng Shui**, Mysticism, Astrology, Painting, Gardening, Spiritual practices, Warfare, and so on.

Read → <u>The Art of War</u>, by Sun Tzu

Chinese medicine is based on observation.
Observe not only with your eyes but also with your heart and soul.

Tao, Dao
Tao is that which has no shape. The Tao cannot be defined. It is the realm from which all things and beings arise and into which everything returns, eventually. It is not a place or space but rather a way of thinking about existence. The Tao knows no division.

*   Everything arises from and dissolves into the Tao
*   Tao is often translated as "The Way"
*   It can also be the beginning and end of all things

As the Tao is beyond grasp of most human minds, ways had to be invented to describe and organize the world we live in. This organization is described by dividing observable phenomena into pairs or elements and by describing their relationship to one another.

Graphic: Yin Yang Complimentary Pairs

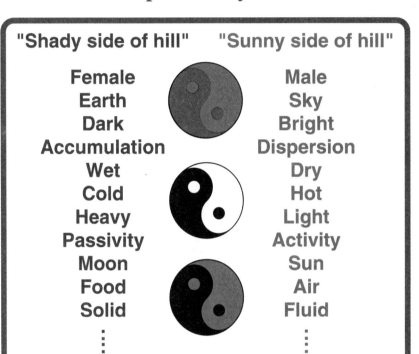

Yin   Yang
Complimentary Pairs

"Shady side of hill"	"Sunny side of hill"
Female	Male
Earth	Sky
Dark	Bright
Accumulation	Dispersion
Wet	Dry
Cold	Hot
Heavy	Light
Passivity	Activity
Moon	Sun
Food	Air
Solid	Fluid
⋮	⋮

Not Complimentary Pairs because these have absolute qualitative/quantitative assessment:

Good/Evil
Superior/Inferior
Big/Small
Apples/Oranges

Not Complimentary Pairs because these don't come in pairs:

Colors
Foods
Pathologies
Racial/Political Groups

Yin/Yang, First Division

Yin/Yang is the concept of complimentary pairs used to compare characteristics or items. Nothing is absolutely Yin nor absolutely Yang. Whether something is Yin or Yang depends on what it is compared to.

Example: Steam is Yang relative to water.
              Steam is Yin relative to air.
In general: The lighter more etheric something is the more Yang it is.
              The heavier or dense something is the more Yin it is.

Yin and Yang are neither is positive or negative, good or bad. The ideal situation arises when Yin mingles with, and balances Yang; when Yin/Yang are plentiful and harmonious.

Yin and Yang can be very general or very specific. They are **quantifiable but not measurable**. Yin and Yang are quantifiable only in terms of **Shi** (excess) and **Xu** (deficiency) relative to one another. Both Shi and Xu of either Yin or Yang will cause disharmony and dis-ease.

Graphic: Yin/Yang Relationships and Expressions

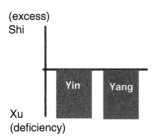

Ideal state: Yin/Yang are balanced and plentiful.
Possible pathology: Yin Yang plentiful but not harmonious.
Example: Hypochondriacs

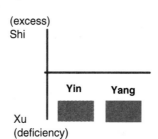

Deficient state: Yin/Yang are balanced but insufficient.
Example: Long time heroin users, starvation, emaciated body without energy,

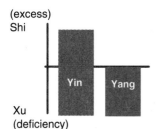

Too much Yin: Person has a big or heavy body but normal energy and drive.
Downside: Maintaining status quo is a constant effort.

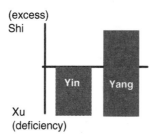

Too much Yang: Person has normal body but is a driven, type A personality, gets things done
Downside: If not properly guided they can be aggressive, destructive.

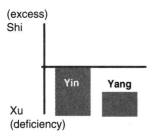

Not enough Yang: Person has normal body but low energy and drive.
Example: Beginning stages of chronic fatigue syndrome, marijuana user

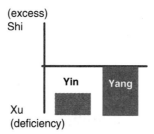

Not enough Yin: Person has thin (lean) body and is high strung, driven.
Example: marathon runners, dancers
Pathology: agitation, insomnia, mental instability

Ideal State
Yin/Yang are plentiful and create each other, control each other, mingle with one another.

Yin/Yang Pathologies
- Yin/Yang imbalance: Plentiful but not harmonious, all kinds of disorders, all at the same time
- Yin deficiency: Dryness, irritation, itching, thirst, skinny, sunken look
- Yang deficiency: No energy, indecisiveness, perpetual cold not warmed by blanket
- Yin Excess: Damp, swollen look, overweight, flabby, cloudy thinking, attached to habits
- Yang excess: Agitated, violent, active, workaholic, tendency to overdue habits, always hot
- Yin/Yang deficiency: Qi deficiency, lethargy, chronic fatigue syndrome, and infertility

Three Treasures

The Three Treasures is a term in TCM that refers to "substances" that make reproduction possible and thus the perpetuation of the species. One who is in possession of all three treasures in sufficient amounts and balance will have no trouble reproducing and thus passing on the Three Treasures.

Graphic: Three Treasures

Shen, Jing, Qi

The three ingredients through which Qi is passed on through the generations

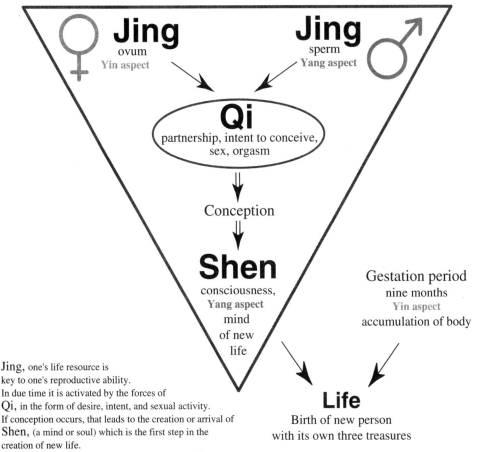

Jing, one's life resource is key to one's reproductive ability. In due time it is activated by the forces of Qi, in the form of desire, intent, and sexual activity. If conception occurs, that leads to the creation or arrival of Shen, (a mind or soul) which is the first step in the creation of new life.

Thus the "Three Treasures" govern procreation.

Shen is the sparkle in the eye, the spirit of human intelligence, clarity, loosely translates as consciousness, drug users will loose or scatter their Shen, thus have dull eyes.
- Shen arrives when male Jing (Yang aspect) and female Jing (Yin aspect) meet through conception.
- Most yang substance in the body, the most etheric.
- Resides in the "Blood" or Xue
- At night it is stored in the Liver, during the day it manifests in the eyes.

Graphic: Jing Stores

Jing can be thought of as a lifetime savings account. Everybody is put into this world with a given amount, some with more, some with less.

Those that manage to hold on to Jing live long and prosper. Those who squander their allotment age faster and die younger.

Jing allows for overall development, vitality, fertility, and maturing.

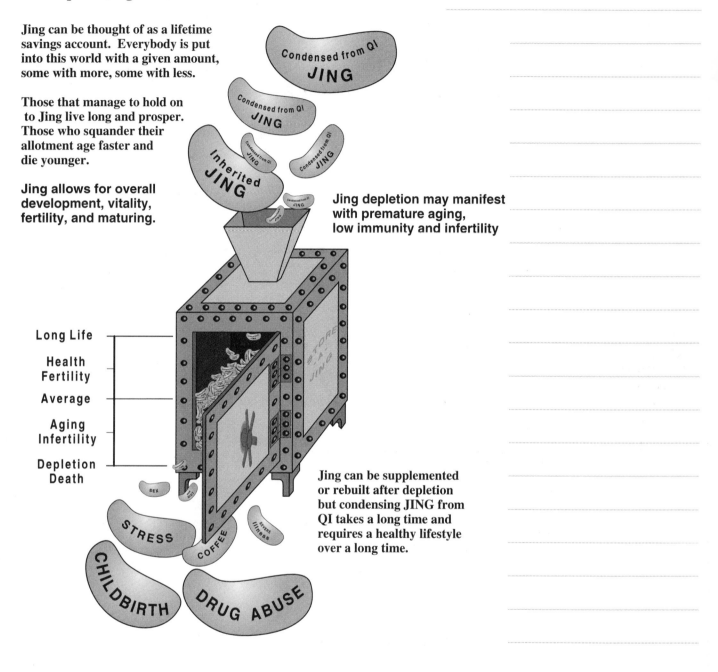

Jing depletion may manifest with premature aging, low immunity and infertility

Long Life

Health
Fertility

Average

Aging
Infertility

Depletion
Death

Jing can be supplemented or rebuilt after depletion but condensing JING from QI takes a long time and requires a healthy lifestyle over a long time.

Jing: The most concentrated store of Qi, is almost tangible, stored in the Kidneys, it is the gift from parents that allows you to draw your first breath, and is the reserve that one can draw on in times of emergency such as famine.

- Easily used up, hard to replace.
- Gradually diminishes throughout life, which is the aging process. When Jing deficient, infertility will result, as well as premature aging.
- Women lose Jing through menstruation and delivery.
  Emphasis for self care is nourishment, even flow.
- Men lose Jing through overwork, ejaculation.
  Emphasis for self care is restraint and regeneration.

Graphic: Jing Balance

JING is required for reproductive health.

Before puberty, JING is insufficient and needs to mature.
During the fertile years it is important to maintain the flow of QI
and an emotional balance.
With progressing age conservation of JING becomes the focus.

How well do you balance your JING expenditures?

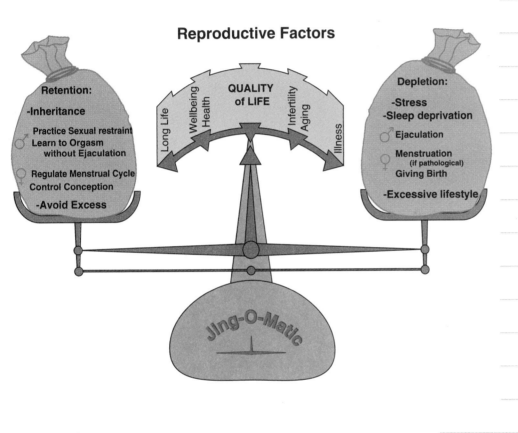

Qi

- Also written as Ki or Chi.
- Without Qi there is no life.
- All schools have the concept of Qi in common.
- Without Qi there is no Chinese medicine.
- Don't translate it into English - there are many words for it (Energy, Breath, life force, ...) and none grasps the concept entirely.
- The term "Energy" particularly will run afoul with individuals that have a physics mind set.

Graphic: Qi v/s Energy

Qi   v/s   Energy

Qi	Energy
aka: "Ki, Chi, Lifeforce"	aka. "Power, Juice, ..."
Defies laws of physics	Defined by laws of physics
Has no unit of measurement	Has units of measurement
Can be assessed but not measured	Can be measured
Only generated by what is alive Can not be genetrated by machines	Can not be genetrated, only converted from one form into another; i.e. thermal, electric, potential, kinetic, chemical, etc.
Moved by acupuncture, massage, movement, intent	Moved by difference in potential
Has various functions in the body	Exists in all forms in the body
Ties together TCM philosophy	Ties together Newtonian physics
Air + Food = Qi	$e = mc^2$

Therefore: Qi is NOT Energy

Although Qi is often translated in casual conversation as "Energy" this is an inappropriate translation when elaborating on the functions and qualities of Qi. Life–force is a better metaphor.

- Qi is the assumed flow of "life force" through the body. This flow follows certain patterns, called meridians, and performs certain functions in the body. It is the foundation of diagnosis, assessment and treatment.
- Qi can be very general or very specific, it is quantifiable but not

measurable.

- Qi in itself may not be perceivable to most but its manifestations can be easily assessed. Similarly, disruptions of the smooth flow of Qi will manifest as pathologies. TCM provides a framework for the assessment of the functions of Qi, as well as treatment modalities that will restore smooth flow, as evidenced by improvement of pathological conditions.

What is "Qi"?

Do Not concern yourself with what Qi is. Experience it through the practice of Tai Qi, Qi Gong or martial arts.

> Feels like a tingle,
> feels like a current,
> feels like heat,
> feels like waking after a great sleep.

Depending on the point of view it is:

- A theoretical construct to help with diagnosis and treatment
- A real force that can be felt, manipulated and manifests in people and all things living
- A cosmic flow of energy between heavens and earth, sometimes in western concepts equated to Ether, Tachions, and other fringe "science" terms
- An energy that can be transmitted over great distances and manifest anywhere
- Many other explanations

When depletion of Qi is stronger than intake, Jing (Constitutional) Qi will fill in and be depleted resulting in premature aging. If expense and intake of Qi are kept in balance, no depletion will results and life force will be strong.

Generation
Qi is generated by Yin and Yang aspects of food and air.

Graphic: Generation of Qi

1. Air enters the lungs,
   Food enters the stomach

2. The Kidney facilitates extraction by
   supplying Qi to the Lung and
   Spleen/Stomach

3. The Lung and Spleen/Stomach thus
   extract pure essences as Air Qi and
   Food Qi and send them to the chest

4. In the chest Air Qi and Food Qi
   combine to form Chest Qi.

5. Chest Qi breaks up into
   its Yin and Yang aspects,
   Nutritive Qi (Ying Qi) and
   Protective (Wei Qi).

7. Wei Qi (Yang aspect) circulates on the
   outside of the body and provides
   protection from pathogens.

8. Ying Qi (Yin aspect) moves inside
   the body and replentishes the Kidneys
   and all Zang/Fu Organs.

Air: (Yang aspect) clean air, long conscious breath; often neglected

Food: (Yin aspect) Gu Qi clean fresh food, no older than 3 days. Eat with the seasons and climate. Food is the most powerful medicine because its taken 3x daily in quantity. Foods are classified for their energy (Qi) producing properties like Herbs.

Generation: Air (Yang aspect) and Food (Yin aspect) form Zheng (Chest) Qi in chest that is undifferentiated. But Zheng Qi splits immediately into Yin and Yang aspects:

Wei: (Protective) Qi (yang aspect), it travels on the outside of the body and circulates on the body surface.

Ying: (Nourishing) Qi (yin aspect, goes on the inside and renourishes organs that need Qi to generate Qi.

Read → Healing with Whole Foods

Functions of Qi

- **Raising**
  – opening eyes
  – raise eyes and smile
  – attitude
  – erection
- **Holding**
  – hold blood inside vessels
  – hold internal organs in place
  – prevent prolapse
  – maintain pregnancy
- **Nourishing**
  – supply organs with Qi and nutrients
  – nourish muscles
- **Protecting**
  – protect from pathogens
  – physical/psychological protection
- **Moving/Warming**
  – move blood and Qi
  – move emotions

Graphic: Five Functions of Qi

Nourishing - keep internal organs supplied with Qi to maintain function, also Ying Qi

Protecting - bodies ability to defend against pathogens, cold, infections, also Wei Qi

Raising - brings Qi to the head, waking up, smiling, counteracts sagging, erection

Holding - keeps things in place, stools, urine, pregnancy, prevents prolapse

Warming/Moving - maintain body temperature, proper distribution of heat

Other Substances Involved
Xue
Xue is the most dense substance in body, most Yin.

Represents two concepts:
1) Physical blood with the same function as in western medicine (blood).
2) Functional concept of "blood" in Chinese medicine, that ties blood into the Qi and meridian context. Xue houses the spirit at night and gives it a home (Blood).

Relationship:
Qi moves Blood
Blood is the mother of Qi

Overhead: Xue, TCM Concept of Blood

Xue combines qualities of both the physical blood and the TCM concepts of Blood

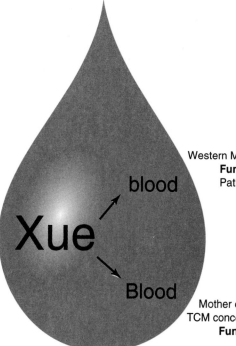

Western Medicine concept, physical blood
    Function: transport Oxygen
    Pathologies: anemia
          not enough blood due to internal/external bleeding
          blood loss due to heavy menstrual cycle

Mother of Qi
TCM concept of Blood, defined by TCM theory
    Function: Houses Shen
        -moves shen into the eyes during Daytime
        -houses Shen in the Liver at night
            Nourish and Lubricate

Pathologies of Xue	Signs +Symptoms
Xue Xu (deficiency)	Paleness, tiredness, flaccid skin, insomnia, craziness when the blood fails to house Shen
Xue Yu (stagnation)	Also called congealed Blood, Bruises, menstrual cramps, sharp stabing pain, tumors, cysts

Jin/Ye

Water Metabolism separated by types of fluids:
> **Jin:** pure fluids moisten eyes, skin, and organs
> **Ye:** impure fluids, metabolic waste, urine, and feces

Water metabolism is primarily the function of the **San Jiao** or **Triple Burner** aka. **Triple Heater**. It is an "Organ" that is not recognized as an organ in western medicine.

• The "Organ" is defined strictly in terms of its functional aspects.
• Used in clinical diagnosis for signs and symptoms of water metabolism and body temperature regulation.
• Includes chest, belly and abdomen as three areas of Triple Burner.

• Organs that govern water metabolism are mostly:
> -Lungs (upper burner/chest) → disseminate pure water and moisten organs and skin.
> -Spleen (middle burner/belly) → separates pure and impure, sends pure up, impure down.
> -Large Intestine (lower burner/abdomen) → reabsorbs water from feces and with the help of the Kidney fire boils (distills) it for recycling in digestion and Lungs.

Graphic: Zang/Fu

Zang (Yin) **Organs**
Solid organs
Process, store pure substances, Qi, Xue

Fu (Yang) **Organs**
Hollow organs
Process, move coarse substances, Food

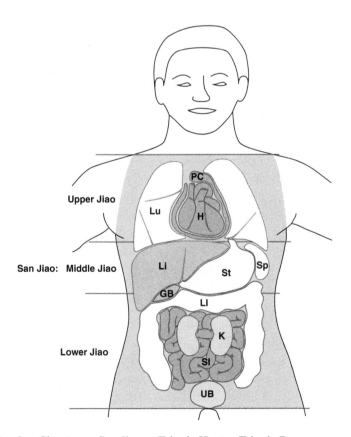

Upper Jiao

San Jiao: Middle Jiao

Lower Jiao

Read → Chapter on San Jiao or Tripple Heater, Tripple Burner

Notes/Questions on San Jiao

Second Division, The Five Elements

The Five Elements are the second level of differentiation that allows for assessment of people, pathologies, nature and related phenomena. Like the Yin/Yang division this is a theoretical construct in which objects, situations and relationships are explored relative to one another.

Now there are five qualities that can be assessed and there are four distinct relationships that tie the theory together. The relationships and expressions are of dynamic nature, thus subject to change. Neither of the Elements is superior to another, the goal is to balance the qualities so that they interact with one another appropriately.

Overhead: Five Elements

Color guide: **Attributes associated with Element**
Yin Organ/Meridian / Yin Organ function
"Chinese Name" / Most active time of day
Yang Organ/Meridian
"Chinese Name" / Most active time

Each Element is associated with one
Yin/Yang Meridian pair, except
Fire which has two pairs

The Five Elements also represent developmental stages in progression and are cyclical in nature, like the seasons in a year, a life span from conception through death and new beginning.

How to read the Five Element Chart
Starting at the center:
*   The Yin Yang Symbol the first differentiation from the Tao in Chinese philosophy.

The first circle:
*   The Five Elements are represented in their corresponding colors and their Element name.

Note: The colors may vary depending on the source.
*   **Fire** is always red.
*   **Earth** is always yellow, although in some charts it may have a tinge to the orange. It is the color of autumn.
*   **Metal** is white on some charts it may be depicted as light blue.
*   **Water** is black, although on some charts it may be dark blue, the color of the night sky.
*   **Wood** is "the color of a dragons skin" as one source puts it, by convention that can be a straight green, or a blue green, or the color of jade.

The arrowheads indicate the relationship between the elements:
*   The **Generating Cycle** follows a clockwise progression.
*   The **Controlling Cycle** also follows a clockwise progression but skips one element; it refers to the positive aspect of that relationship. When one element becomes overbearing on another the result is **Over Control**. This cycle follows the same progression as the controlling cycle but is pathological.
*   The **Insulting Cycle** runs counter clockwise and always refers to a pathological situation between the elements.

*   Moving outward, the Yin/Yang paired channels are listed. The Yin channel is in blue, the Yang channel is in red. Each element has one pair except for the Fire Element that contains two pairs: Heart/Small Intestine and San Jiao/Pericardium.

*   Under the English channel name is the Chinese name in Pin Yin and the time of day when the channel is most active Next to the Yin channel (in blue) are the qualities associated with its function.

*   Above the English channel name is the essential function of the organ according to Chinese medical theory.

*   On the outside of each segment (in black) finally are the basic correspondences as they refer to each of the Five Elements. This list is by no means complete but rather serves to illustrate the basic relation to natural phenomena.

Interactions

Generating: Fire leaves ashes -> creates earth
Metal is found in the ground (earth)
Water condenses on metal
Water makes wood grow
Wood feeds fire

Graphic: Five Element Interactions (1)

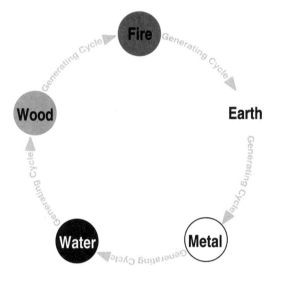

Generating Cycle:

- Positive Cycle
- Clockwise progression
- One element leads to the generation of the next
- All elements in balance

Pathology:
- Failure to generate
- Elements out of balance

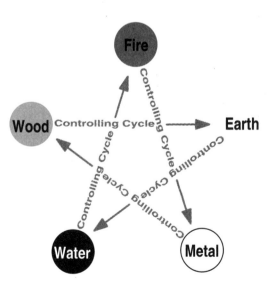

Controlling Cycle:

- Positive Cycle
- Clockwise progression
- Controlling element skips adjacent element
- Keeps generating cycle in check
- All elements in balance

Pathology:
- Failure to control
- Too much control (Overcontrol)

Controlling: Fire (heat) makes metal pliable
Metal trims wood (lawnmover)
Wood holds Earth in place
Earth holds water in channels and dams
Water cools fire (heat)

Over controlling: Fire melts metal
Metal cuts wood
Wood displaces earth
Earth soaks up water
Water puts out fire

Graphic: Five Element Interactions (2)

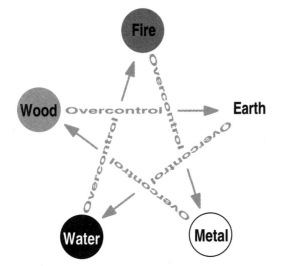

Overcontrol Cycle:

- Negative Cycle
- Clockwise progression
  (same as **Control cycle**)
- Overcontrolling element skips
  adjacent element

Pathology:
- Overcontrol prevents Generation
- Throws elements out of balance

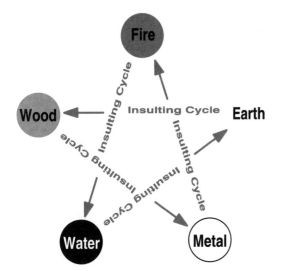

Insulting Cycle:

- Negative Cycle
- Counter clockwise progression
- Insulting element skips previous element

Pathology:
- Insulting cycle leads to failure
  of Generation cycle
- Drains insulted element
- Throws elements out of balance

Insulting: Metal can put out fire
Fire can evaporate water
Water can wash away earth
Earth can crush wood
Wood dulls metal

Each elements have assigned qualities: Emotions, sounds, growth stages,
foods, animals, seasons, colors etc.

Arrangements

Graphic: Possible Five Element Arrangements

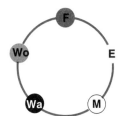

- Most frequently seen arrangement.
- Elements are arranged in generating fashion with Fire in highest position. (Flames flicker upward)
- In term of seasonal arrangements Earth is the Indian Summer from early September into November.

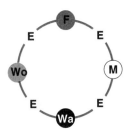

- Sometimes seen in this arrangement, especially when referring to sesonal changes.
- Each of the main four seasons end with a quiet period that indicates change into the next.

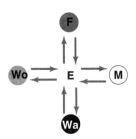

- This arrangement is popular when using Earth as the center.
- Fire rises.
- Water disappears below ground.
- Wood rises (through growth).
- Metal sinks.

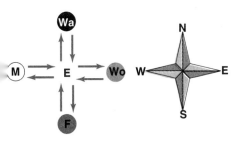

- This arrangement is popular when refering to the climatic conditions. (Northern hemisphere only)
- In the North it is cold, wintery, and in the South it is hot and sunny,
- Positions of Metal and Wood result from the progression between the elements.

Play the Five Element Party Game.
Find associations within the Five Elements that apply to yourself or your
friends, find out what the dynamic of your relationship is. These are some of
the phrases that might give away a persons Element association.

Overhead: Element Date

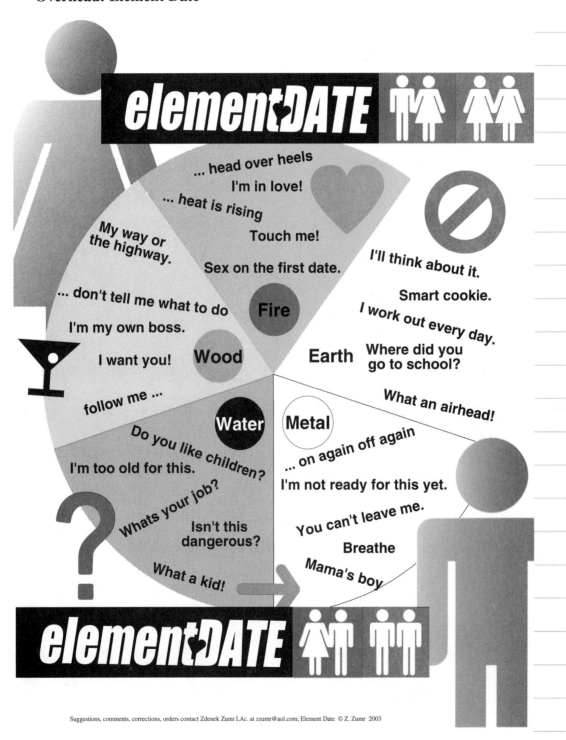

Feng Shui

One popular application of the Five Element theory is Feng Shui, or the divination of location and space. This can be applied to interior design, architecture, and particularly, landscaping. A garden is arranged so that the Five Elements are in harmony with one another.

- **Fire**: Bright spaces with light colored rocks to reflect the sunlight, white washed walls or light loving plants
- **Earth**: Ground cover such as moss, short grasses or unplanted areas covered in mulch
- **Metal**: Sculptures, bells, castings, also buildings and archways
- **Water**: Ponds, waterfalls, fountains
- **Wood**: Trees and tall shrubs

Graphic: Geomancy Compass

Instrument used in the art and practice of Feng Shui

Utilized to this day to divine the best arrangement of objects according to the cardinal directions, Yin/Yang, The five Elements and the flow of Qi, so that they are in harmony with one another and human nature.

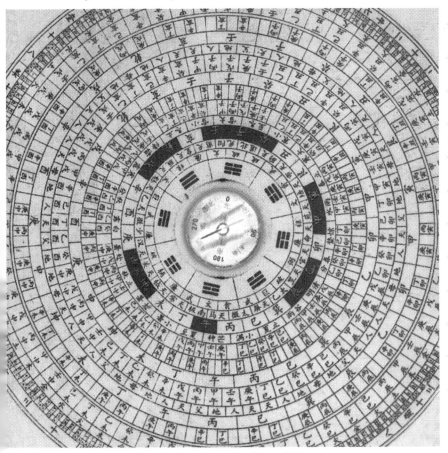

Antique ivory carving from China.

Feng Shui was also used in ancient times in warfare in setting up a battle field in ones favor.

Read → Sun Tzu: The Art of War

Notes

Third Division, 12 Meridians

At this point we are leaving general aspects of Chinese philosophy and move specifically into medicinal aspects of Qi flow.

There are in Chinese medicine 12 Organ Channels or Primary Meridians, Vessels, Pathways, etc.

- They are divided into 6 Yin and 6 Yang and follow several patterns on the body that should make it easy to remember:

	YIN	YANG
FIRE	Heart, Pericardium	Small Intestine, San Jiao
EARTH	Spleen	Stomach
METAL	Lung	Large Intestine
WATER	Kidney	Urinary Bladder
WOOD	Liver	Gall Bladde

Graphic: Meridian Flow

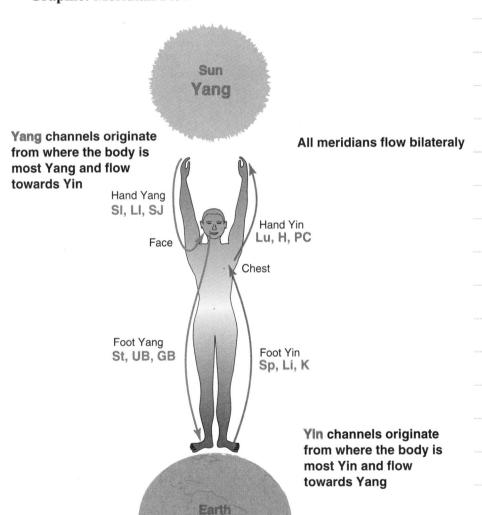

Sun
Yang

Yang channels originate from where the body is most Yang and flow towards Yin

All meridians flow bilateraly

Hand Yang
SI, LI, SJ

Hand Yin
Lu, H, PC

Face

Chest

Foot Yang
St, UB, GB

Foot Yin
Sp, Li, K

Yin channels originate from where the body is most Yin and flow towards Yang

Earth
Yin

- Yang channels originate where the body is more Yang in comparison to its ending. Hand Yang originate in the finger tips and end in the face.
- Yin channels originate where the body is more Yin in comparison to its ending. Hand Yin originate in the chest and end in the finger tips.

Another way to group the channels is according to where they flow. There are six meridians that start or end in the hands and six meridians that start or end in the feet.

	HAND	FOOT
YIN	Pericardium, Heart, Lung	Spleen, Kidney, Liver
YANG	San Jiao, Small Intestine, Large Intestine	Stomach, Urinary Bladder Gall Bladder

Thus each meridian can be characterized as either HAND-YIN, HAND-YANG, FOOT-YIN, or FOOT-YANG. The characterizations determine where the meridians begin and end.

There are 24 hours in a day and 12 meridians, it follows that each meridian will have a peak flow for two hours per day. The meridians carry Qi sequentially and follow predetermined pathways that cover the body. To follow the flow of Qi through the body in a 24-hour period, trace the spiral in clockwise direction with a finger.

Graphic: Yin Yang Clock

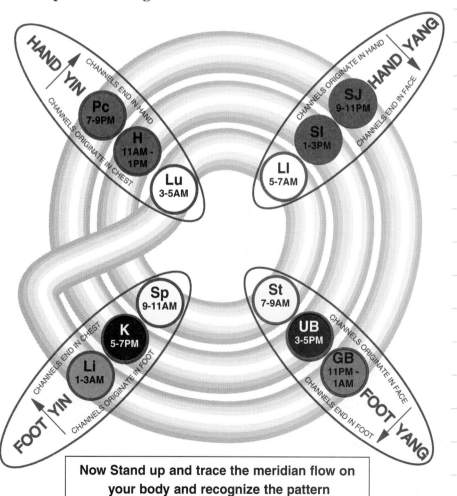

Now Stand up and trace the meridian flow on
your body and recognize the pattern

The principle pathway (Hand Yin → Hand Yang → Foot Yang → Foot Yin back to Hand Yin) repeats itself three times.

Every meridian has an organ associated with it. The Chinese medical organs are functional concepts that include some of the western medicinal functions but also refer to their involvement in manufacturing Qi.

* Although the meridians carry the names of internal organs, the Chinese medicine organs are NOT the same as organs in western medicine .*

A person that had their spleen or gall bladder removed will still have Spleen or Gall Bladder meridian as well as related organ pathologies.

By convention organ names that are capitalized will refer to the Chinese medicine concept and names that are in lower case will refere to the western medicine organ.

Qi is flowing from one meridian to another. The end point of a meridian is never too far from the beginning point of the successive meridian. On a 24 hour time clock this is the progression of the meridians in the day.

Graphic: 24 Hour Progression

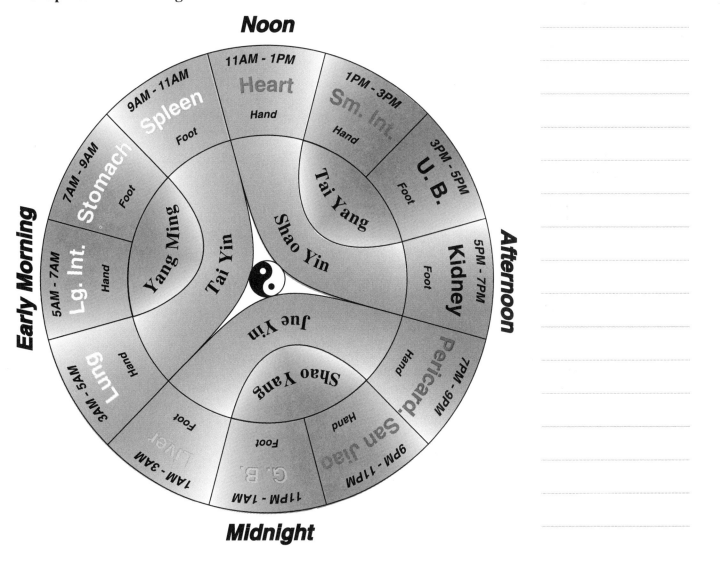

Zang/Fu

The Zang/Fu is the study of internal organ function in Chinese medicine. Similarly to the meridian concept, this system includes the actual physical organs but also includes Chinese medicine concepts of organs as well as emotional and psychological manifestations of organ disorders.

Graphic: Zang/Fu

Zang (Yin) **Organs**
Solid organs
Process, store pure substances, Qi, Xue

Fu (Yang) **Organs**
Hollow organs
Process, move coarse substances,

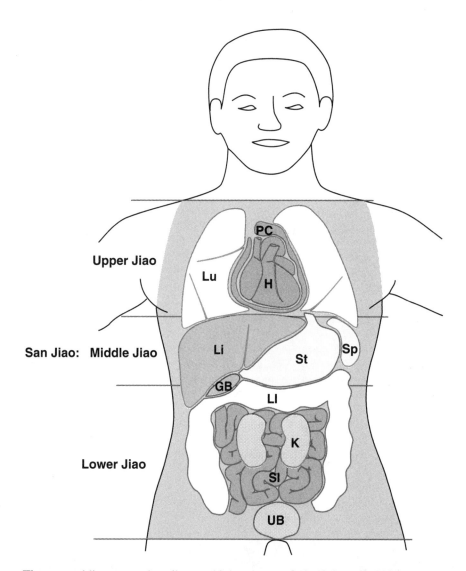

Upper Jiao

San Jiao: Middle Jiao

Lower Jiao

PC
Lu
H
Li
St
Sp
GB
LI
K
SI
UB

Thus a meridian name describes multiple aspects of physiology in Chinese medicine. The name relates to the flow of Qi and related pathologies of Qi, it also describes the Zang/Fu organ function as well as related emotional states. Finally it describes a relation to the actual physical organ/function as described in western medicine. In practice there is no distinction between the various aspects since a good TCM practitioner will consider all aspects of a patients health before beginning treatment.

Graphic: Physical Conceptual aspects of TCM

In TCM, any given organ name describes not only the physical (western medicine) organ but also names the associated meridian of that organ, the TCM Zang/Fu concept relating to the physical organ, as well as the emotional and spiritual components associated with that organ.

By convention if the name is written in lower case it describes the physical organ, if the name is written in upper case it refers to the TCM concept/meridian

Heart for example includes:

a.) heart - physical heart that pumps blood

H1

H9

b.) Heart Meridian (H) - the pathway where Qi flows and where heart (physical) or Heart (TCM), (emotional) pathologies may manifest

c.) Zang/Fu Heart - covers physiological aspects of TCM theory - move Blood, **Xue**

d.) Emotional Heart - expressing, perceiving emotions, esp. love, also within the **Five Elements** Heart is associated with **Fire** whose emotion is **Joy**, thus its healthy expression is governed by heart

The TCM aspects of organ pathologies are in general not in conflict with western medical understanding of the organs, TCM simply adds more layers through which diagnosis is possible.

Notes

Meridians
Time to get the washable markers out!

Trace the meridians as they flow in timely progression.

Make sure to mark   -Direction of flow

                       -Yin or Yang

                       -Beginning/End

                       -Special landmark points

                       -Interesting points for the massage practitioner (page 73)

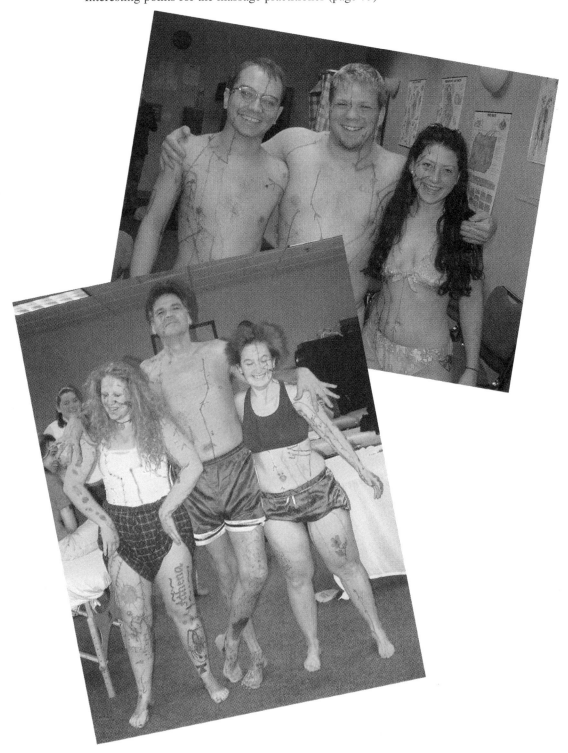

Graphic: Lung Meridian

Lung (Lu), Hand Yin ▲ Meridian, Zang Organ,

Metal Element, Yang compliment is Large Intestine (LI)

Flows from chest to hand from 3 AM to 5 AM

Hand Tai-Yin paired with Foot Tai-Yin of Spleen (Sp)

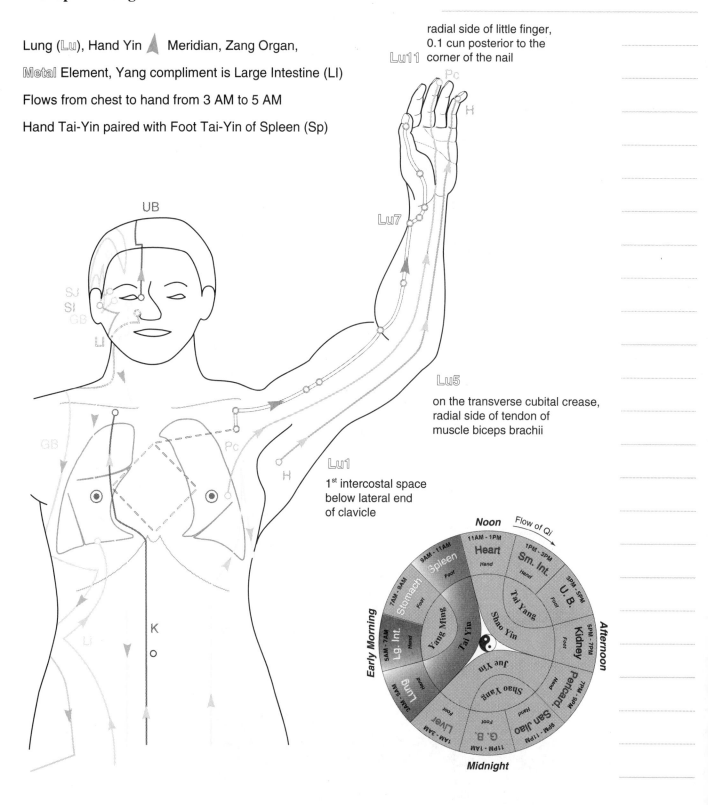

radial side of little finger,
0.1 cun posterior to the
corner of the nail

Lu11

Lu7

Lu5

on the transverse cubital crease,
radial side of tendon of
muscle biceps brachii

Lu1

1st intercostal space
below lateral end
of clavicle

Lungs: Rule Qi → creation, generation, and movement
- Moisten organs and skin → dry skin, clamy skin, eczema.
- "Before you can bring in the new you have to let go of the old" shallow breathing, issues of attachment, letting go.

Graphic: Zang/Fu Syndromes: Lung

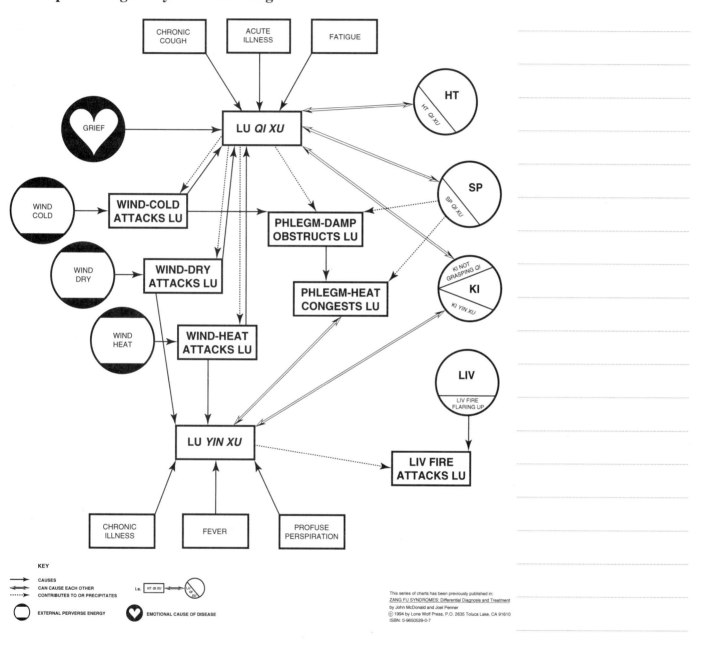

KEY

→ CAUSES
⇒ CAN CAUSE EACH OTHER
┈┈▶ CONTRIBUTES TO OR PRECIPITATES
◯ EXTERNAL PERVERSE ENERGY
♥ EMOTIONAL CAUSE OF DISEASE

i.e. HT QI XU ⇐ LU QI XU

This series of charts has been previously published in:
ZANG FU SYNDROMES: Differential Diagnosis and Treatment
by John McDonald and Joel Penner
© 1994 by Lone Wolf Press, P.O. 2635 Toluca Lake, CA 91610
ISBN: 0-9650529-0-7

This collection of flow charts and graphs was published in the book:
ZANG FU SYNDROMES: DIFFERENTIAL DIAGNOSIS AND TREATMENT
by John McDonald and Joel Penner
published by Lone Wolf Press, P.O. 2635 Toluca Lake, CA 91610
ISBN: 0-9650529-0-7
www.americandragon.com

Graphic: Large Intestine Meridian

Large Intestine (LI), Hand Yang ▼ Meridian, Fu Organ,

Metal Element, Yin compliment is Lung (Lu)

Flows from hand to face from 5 AM to 7 AM

Hand Yang-Ming paired with
    Foot Yang-Ming of Stomach (St)

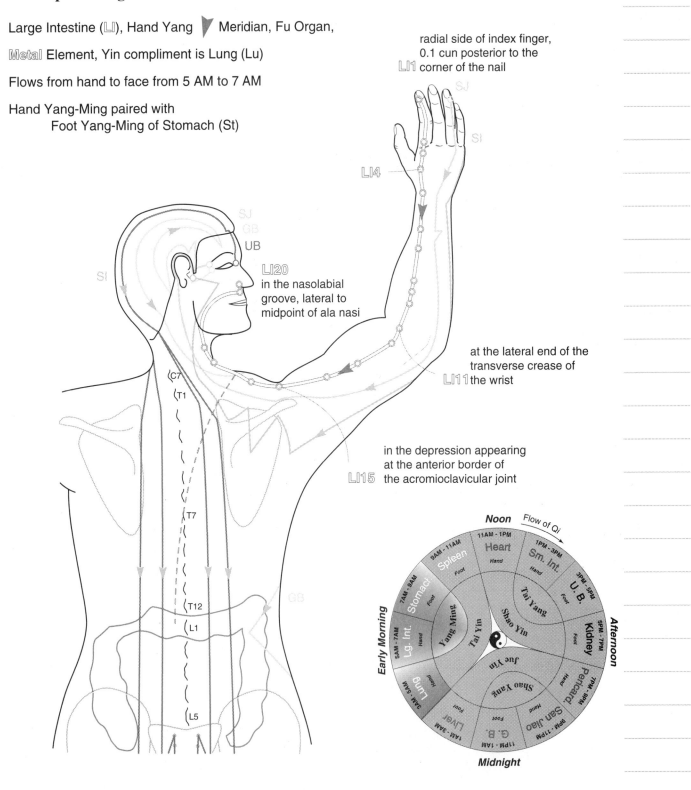

radial side of index finger,
0.1 cun posterior to the
LI1 corner of the nail

LI20
in the nasolabial
groove, lateral to
midpoint of ala nasi

at the lateral end of the
transverse crease of
LI11 the wrist

in the depression appearing
at the anterior border of
LI15 the acromioclavicular joint

Large Intestine: Reabsorption of water, form the feces and "let go of the old".

Graphic: Zang/Fu Syndromes: Large Intestine

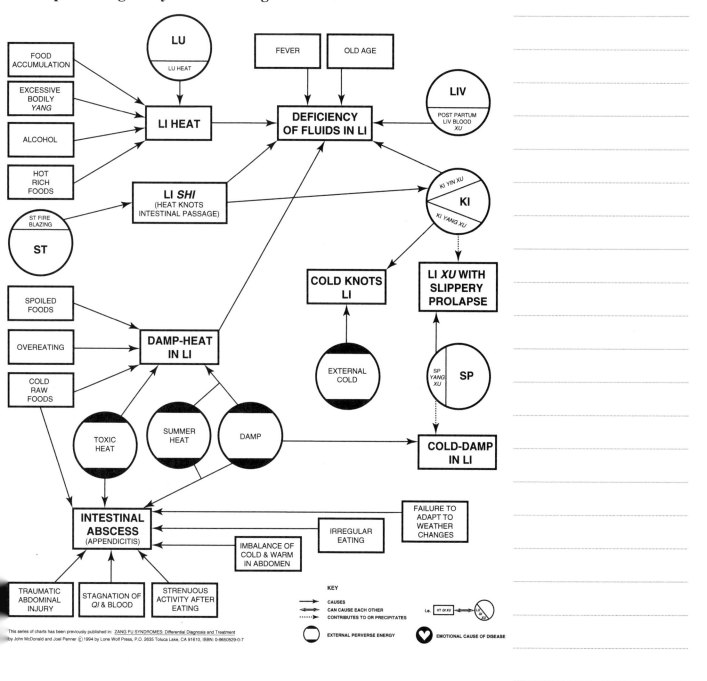

This series of charts has been previously published in: ZANG FU SYNDROMES: Differential Diagnosis and Treatment by John McDonald and Joel Penner © 1994 by Lone Wolf Press, P.O. 2635 Toluca Lake, CA 91610, ISBN: 0-9650529-0-7

Graphic: Stomach Meridian

Stomach Meridian

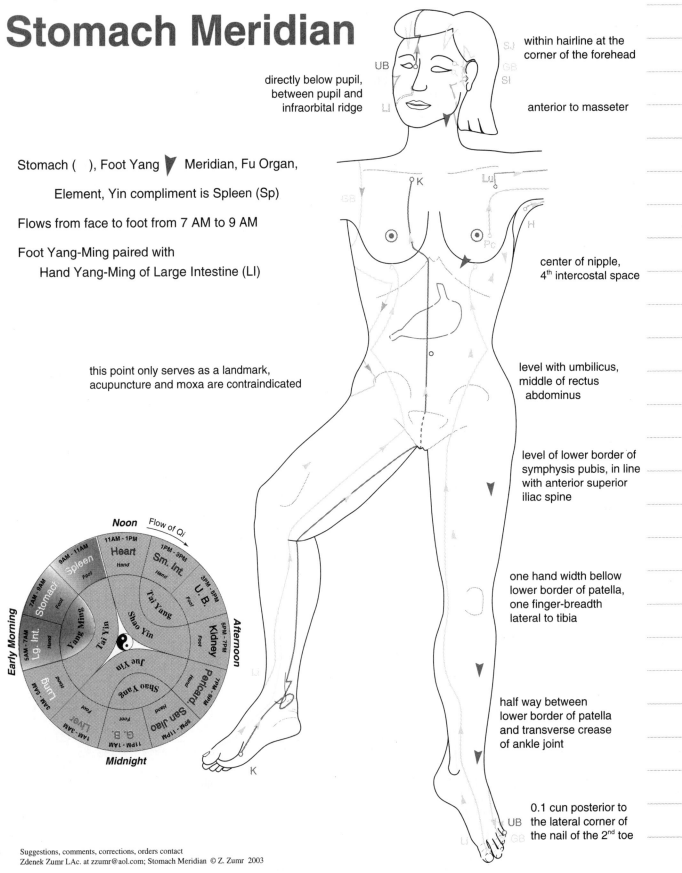

Stomach (   ), Foot Yang ▼ Meridian, Fu Organ,

Element, Yin compliment is Spleen (Sp)

Flows from face to foot from 7 AM to 9 AM

Foot Yang-Ming paired with
 Hand Yang-Ming of Large Intestine (LI)

this point only serves as a landmark,
acupuncture and moxa are contraindicated

within hairline at the
corner of the forehead

directly below pupil,
between pupil and
infraorbital ridge

anterior to masseter

center of nipple,
4th intercostal space

level with umbilicus,
middle of rectus
abdominus

level of lower border of
symphysis pubis, in line
with anterior superior
iliac spine

one hand width bellow
lower border of patella,
one finger-breadth
lateral to tibia

half way between
lower border of patella
and transverse crease
of ankle joint

0.1 cun posterior to
the lateral corner of
the nail of the 2nd toe

Noon

Flow of Qi

Midnight

Suggestions, comments, corrections, orders contact
Zdenek Zumr LAc. at zzumr@aol.com; Stomach Meridian © Z. Zumr 2003

Yang organs, receive and excrete

(also called the hollow Organs, separate pure and impure)

- The Yang organs essentially comprise the digestive tract including the urinary bladder and "San Jiao" also called Triple Heater or Triple Burner. Theit function closely relates to the western understanding of organ function.
- In Chinese medicine Yang organs are used for the treatment of more physical signs and symptoms, imbalances, whereas Yin organs are more used to treat energetic imbalances.

Stomach: Food is broken down and the "pure substances" are separated and sent to the Spleen.

Graphic: Zang/Fu Syndromes: Stomach

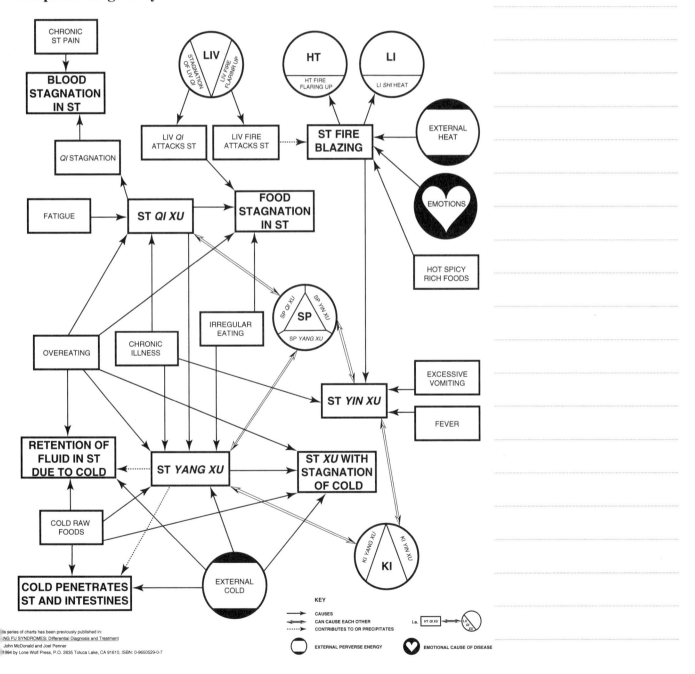

is series of charts has been previously published in:
NG FU SYNDROMES: Differential Diagnosis and Treatment
John McDonald and Joel Penner
1994 by Lone Wolf Press, P.O. 2635 Toluca Lake, CA 91610, ISBN: 0-9650529-0-7

Graphic: Spleen Meridian

Spleen Meridian

Spleen (   ), Foot Yin 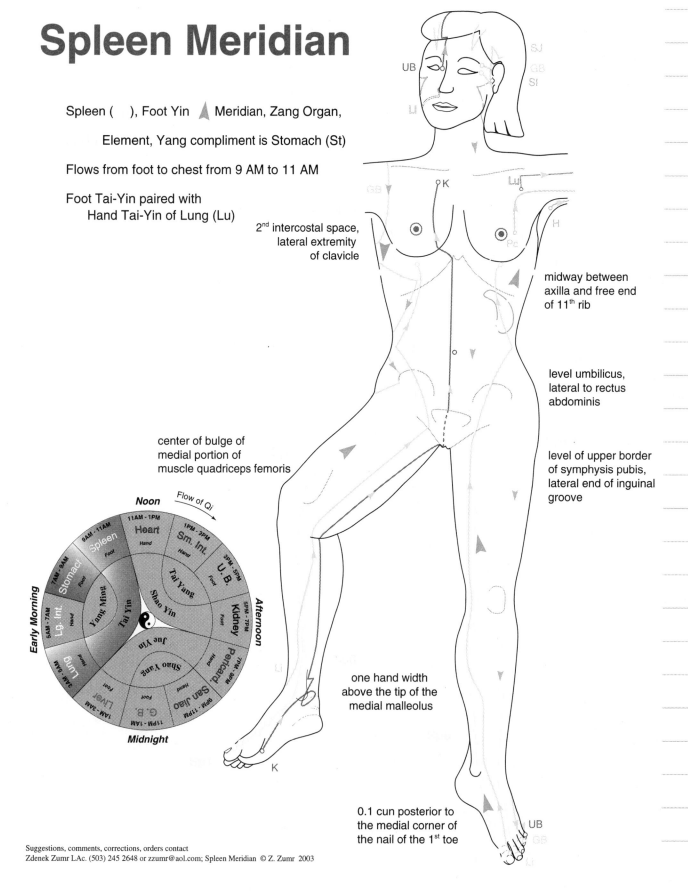 Meridian, Zang Organ,

Element, Yang compliment is Stomach (St)

Flows from foot to chest from 9 AM to 11 AM

Foot Tai-Yin paired with
Hand Tai-Yin of Lung (Lu)

2nd intercostal space,
lateral extremity
of clavicle

midway between
axilla and free end
of 11th rib

level umbilicus,
lateral to rectus
abdominis

center of bulge of
medial portion of
muscle quadriceps femoris

level of upper border
of symphysis pubis,
lateral end of inguinal
groove

one hand width
above the tip of the
medial malleolus

0.1 cun posterior to
the medial corner of
the nail of the 1st toe

Suggestions, comments, corrections, orders contact
Zdenek Zumr LAc. (503) 245 2648 or zzumr@aol.com; Spleen Meridian © Z. Zumr 2003

Spleen: Transformation & transportation of food
- "Good Spleen - good health"
- Deriving Qi from food → chronic fatigue
- Generation of blood, Blood → maintain Xue, i.e. fertility, manifests in the Lips: Red, full lips signal fertility.

Graphic: Zang/Fu Syndromes: Spleen

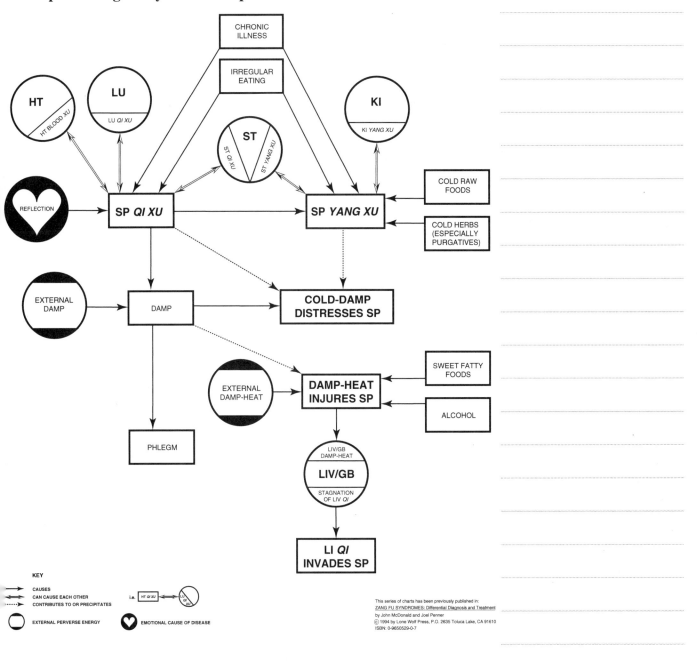

This series of charts has been previously published in:
ZANG FU SYNDROMES: Differential Diagnosis and Treatment
by John McDonald and Joel Penner
© 1994 by Lone Wolf Press, P.O. 2635 Toluca Lake, CA 91610
ISBN: 0-9650529-0-7

Graphic: Heart Meridian

Heart (**H**), Hand Yin ▲ Meridian, Zang Organ,

Fire Element, Yang compliment is Small Intestine (SI)

Flows from chest to hand from 11 AM to 1 PM

Hand Shao-Yin paired with Foot Shao-Yin of Kidney (K)

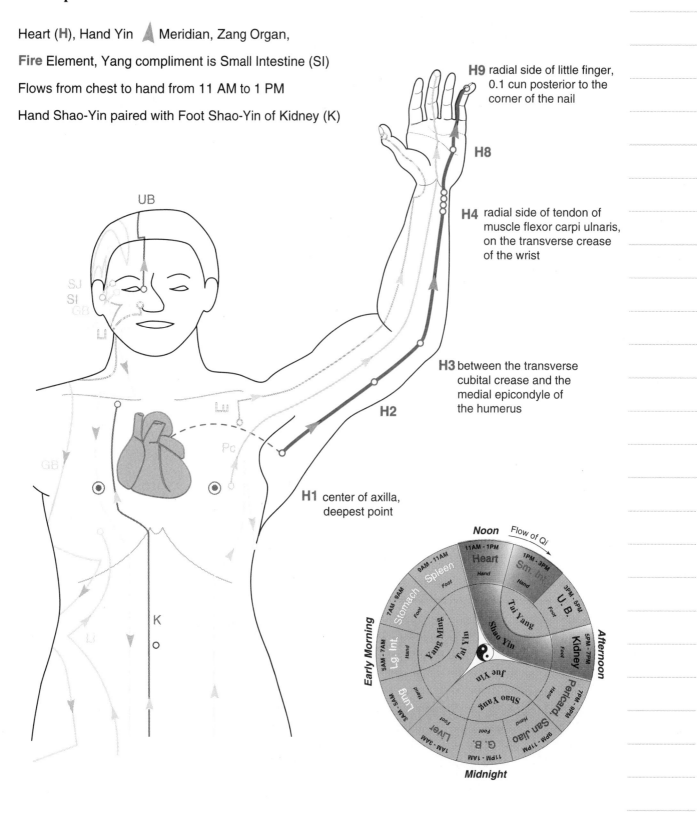

H9 radial side of little finger, 0.1 cun posterior to the corner of the nail

H8

H4 radial side of tendon of muscle flexor carpi ulnaris, on the transverse crease of the wrist

H3 between the transverse cubital crease and the medial epicondyle of the humerus

H2

H1 center of axilla, deepest point

Yin, pure organs
(Also called the full Organs) produce, transform, regulate, and store fundamental substances, Qi, Shen, Blood, Jing, Fluids versus Yang organs (also called the hollow Organs) that receive, break down, absorb, transport, and excrete food.

Heart: (Yin), rules the Blood
- Manifests in face → facial expressions, sunny, grumpy
- Governs Shen → peace of mind, insanity, nightmares
- Check tip of tongue: If red or peeled that would indicate Heart issues, aggravation.

Graphic: Zang/Fu Syndromes: Heart

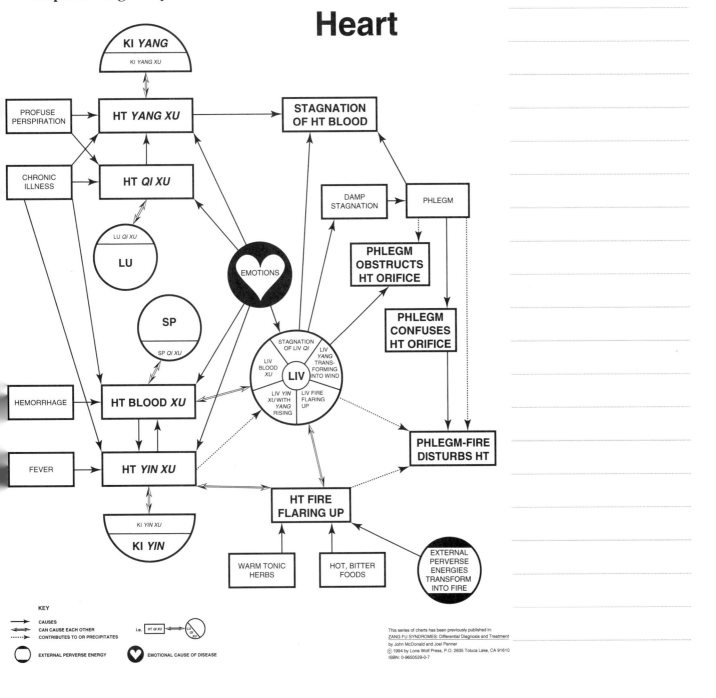

Heart

This series of charts has been previously published in:
ZANG FU SYNDROMES: Differential Diagnosis and Treatment
by John McDonald and Joel Penner
© 1994 by Lone Wolf Press, P.O. 2635 Toluca Lake, CA 91610
ISBN: 0-9650529-0-7

Graphic: Small Intestine Meridian

Small Intestine (**SI**), Hand Yang ▼ Meridian, Fu Organ,

Fire Element, Yin compliment is Heart (H)

Flows from hand to face from 1 PM to 3 PM

Hand Tai-Yang paired with
    Foot Tai-Yang of Urinary Bladder (UB)

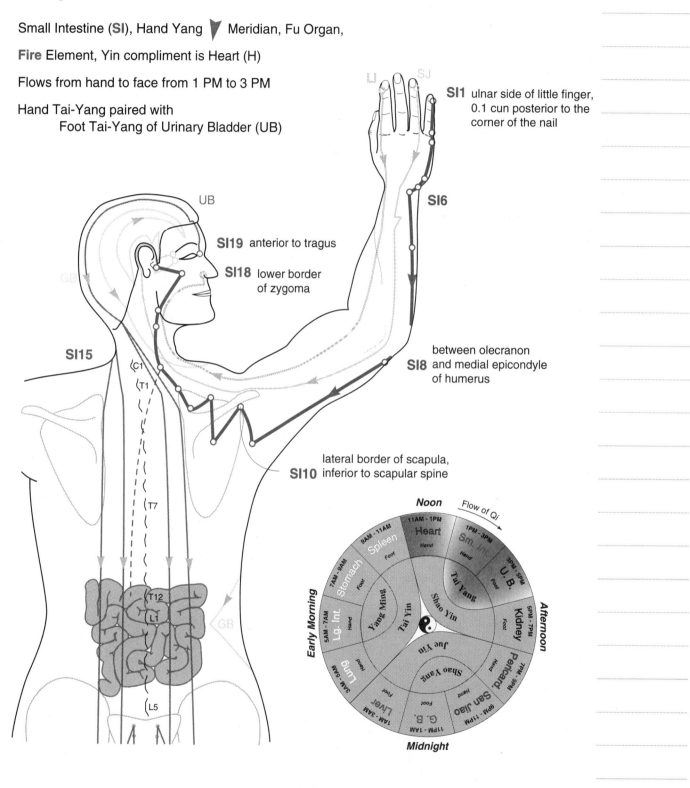

SI1 ulnar side of little finger,
0.1 cun posterior to the
corner of the nail

SI6

SI19 anterior to tragus

SI18 lower border
of zygoma

SI15

SI8 between olecranon
and medial epicondyle
of humerus

SI10 lateral border of scapula,
inferior to scapular spine

Small Intestine: Further break down of foods, "pure substances" are separated and send to the Spleen, turbid fluids are extracted and send to Kidney / Urinary Bladder.

Graphic: Zang/Fu Syndromes: Small Intestine

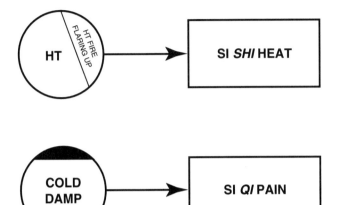

[SI *XU* COLD: SEE SP *YANG XU*]

Graphic: Urinary Bladder Meridian

Urinary Bladder Meridian

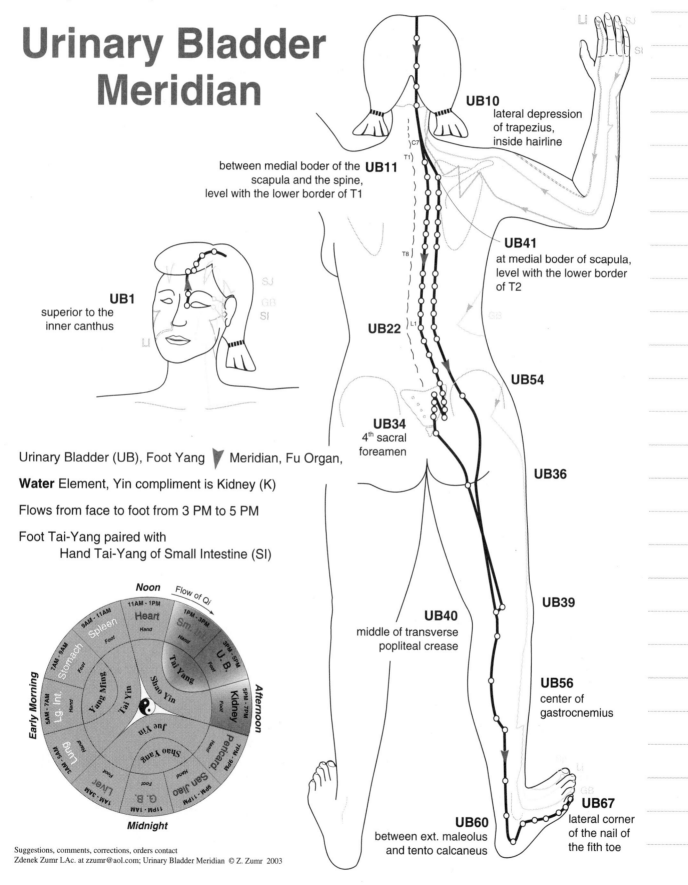

UB10 lateral depression of trapezius, inside hairline

between medial boder of the **UB11** scapula and the spine, level with the lower border of T1

UB41 at medial boder of scapula, level with the lower border of T2

UB22

UB1 superior to the inner canthus

UB54

UB34 4th sacral foreamen

UB36

Urinary Bladder (UB), Foot Yang ▼ Meridian, Fu Organ,

Water Element, Yin compliment is Kidney (K)

Flows from face to foot from 3 PM to 5 PM

Foot Tai-Yang paired with Hand Tai-Yang of Small Intestine (SI)

UB39

UB40 middle of transverse popliteal crease

UB56 center of gastrocnemius

UB67 lateral corner of the nail of the fith toe

UB60 between ext. maleolus and tento calcaneus

Urinary Bladder: Collect and store urine "turbid fluid", Ye fluids.
* Longest channel in the body.
* Channel with the most points.
* Contains Back Shu (diagnostic) points of all organs.

Graphic: Zang/Fu Syndromes: Urinary Bladder

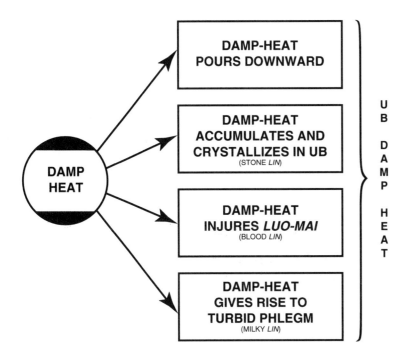

[UB *QI XU*: SEE KI *QI* NOT CONSOLIDATED]

Graphic: Kidney Meridian

Kidney Meridian

Kidney (**Ki**), Foot Yin ▲ Meridian, Zang Organ,

Water Element, Yang compliment is Urinary Bladder (UB)

Flows from foot to chest from 5 PM to 7 PM

Foot Shao-Yin paired with
    Hand Shao-Yin of Heart (H)

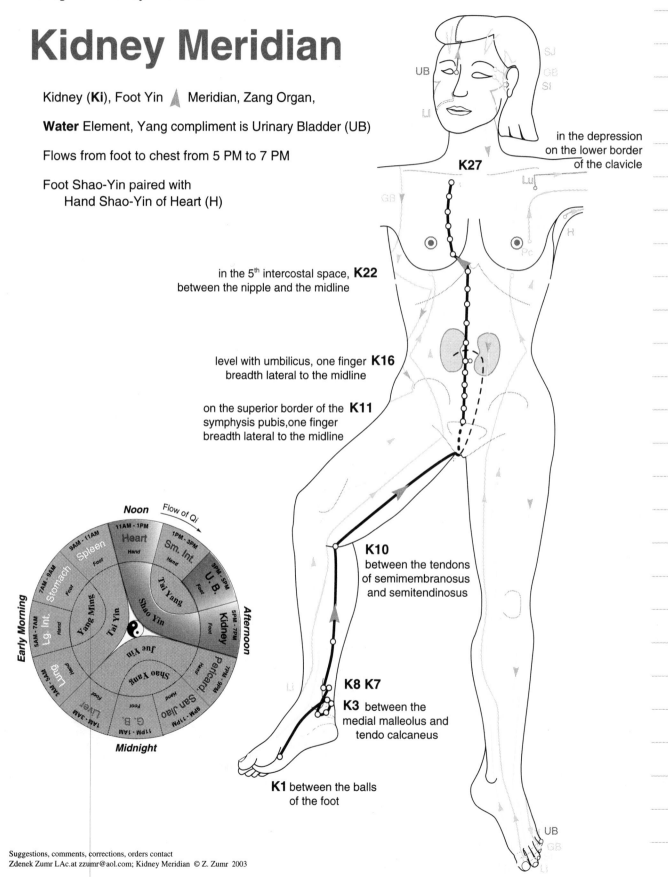

in the depression
on the lower border
of the clavicle

K27

in the 5th intercostal space, **K22**
between the nipple and the midline

level with umbilicus, one finger **K16**
breadth lateral to the midline

on the superior border of the **K11**
symphysis pubis, one finger
breadth lateral to the midline

Noon   Flow of Qi

K10
between the tendons
of semimembranosus
and semitendinosus

K8 K7

K3 between the
medial malleolus and
tendo calcaneus

K1 between the balls
of the foot

Suggestions, comments, corrections, orders contact
Zdenek Zumr LAc.at zzumr@aol.com; Kidney Meridian © Z. Zumr 2003

Kidney: Govern cycle of fertility, maturation, life.
- Root of life, base for activity of all other organs, depend on all other organs for support.
- Low back pain effect of aging → sign of depletion of Jing
- Governs water → edema, frequent urination
- Aging is normal - normal function of Jing (act your age) if aging is resisted → indication of Jing disharmony.
- If aging is premature, hair, teeth, hearing, bone loss etc. → may be indication of Jing insufficiency / disharmony.

Graphic: Zang/Fu Syndromes: Kidney

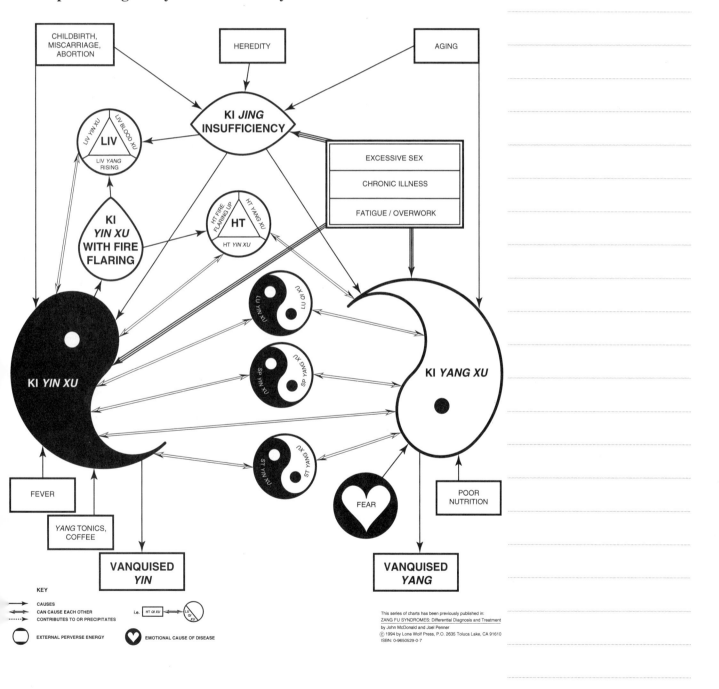

Graphic: Pericardium Meridian

Pericarduim (**Pc**), Hand Yin ▲ Meridian, Zang Organ,

Fire Element, Yang compliment is San Jiao (SJ)

Flows from chest to hand from 7 PM to 9 PM

Hand Jue-Yin paired with Foot Jue-Yin of Liver (Li)

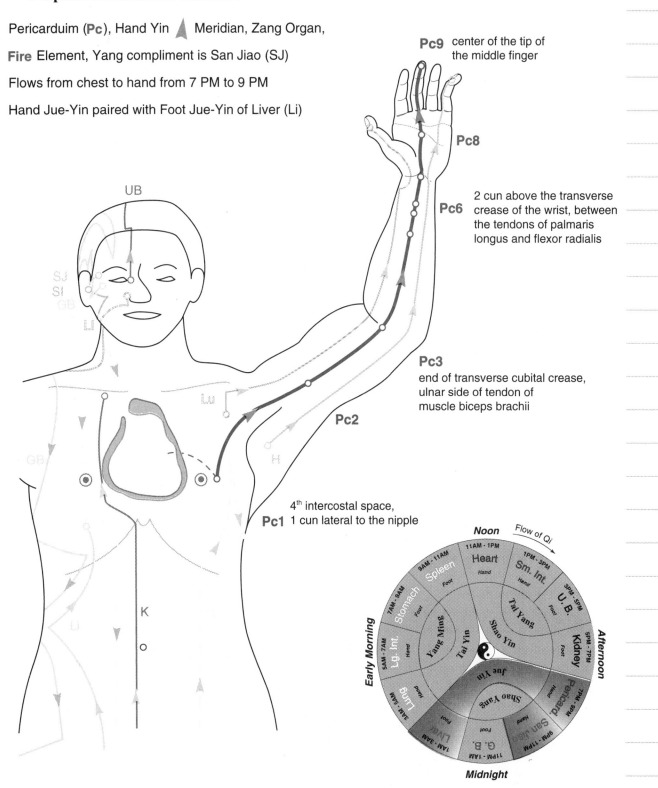

Pc9 center of the tip of the middle finger

Pc8

Pc6 2 cun above the transverse crease of the wrist, between the tendons of palmaris longus and flexor radialis

Pc3 end of transverse cubital crease, ulnar side of tendon of muscle biceps brachii

Pc2

Pc1 4th intercostal space, 1 cun lateral to the nipple

Pathologies between Heart and Pericardium are very similar. The Pericardium is the protector of the heart/Heart - as such pathologies manifest first in the pericardium and then progress into the heart/Heart.

Graphic: San Jiao Meridian

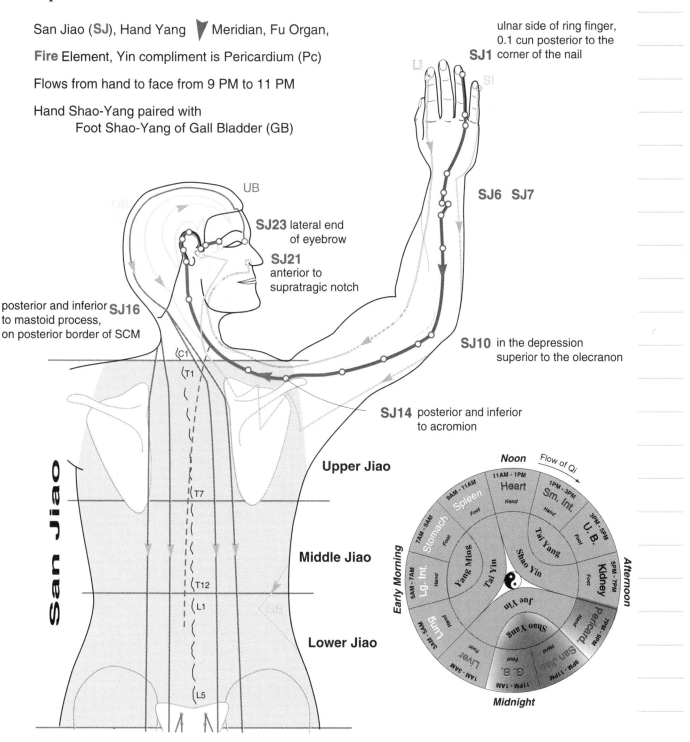

San Jiao (**SJ**), Hand Yang ▼ Meridian, Fu Organ,

Fire Element, Yin compliment is Pericardium (Pc)

Flows from hand to face from 9 PM to 11 PM

Hand Shao-Yang paired with
    Foot Shao-Yang of Gall Bladder (GB)

SJ1 ulnar side of ring finger, 0.1 cun posterior to the corner of the nail

SJ6 SJ7

SJ23 lateral end of eyebrow

SJ21 anterior to supratragic notch

posterior and inferior **SJ16** to mastoid process, on posterior border of SCM

SJ10 in the depression superior to the olecranon

SJ14 posterior and inferior to acromion

Upper Jiao

Middle Jiao

Lower Jiao

San Jiao

Noon — Flow of Qi

The San Jiao exists merely as a functional aspect of water metabolism. It is comprised of the organs in the Three Jiao:,
Upper Jiao , primarily the Lung (dispersing water mist)
Middle Jiao, Spleen and Stomach (boiling water)
Lower Jiao, Large Intestine. (collecting waste water), Kidney (separating)

Graphic: Gall Bladder Meridian

Gall Bladder Meridian

Gall Bladder (**GB**), Foot Yang ▼ Meridian, Fu Organ,

Wood Element, Yin compliment is Liver (Li)

Flows from face to foot from 11 PM to 1 AM

Foot Shao-Yang paired with

 Hand Shao-Yang of San Jiao (SJ)

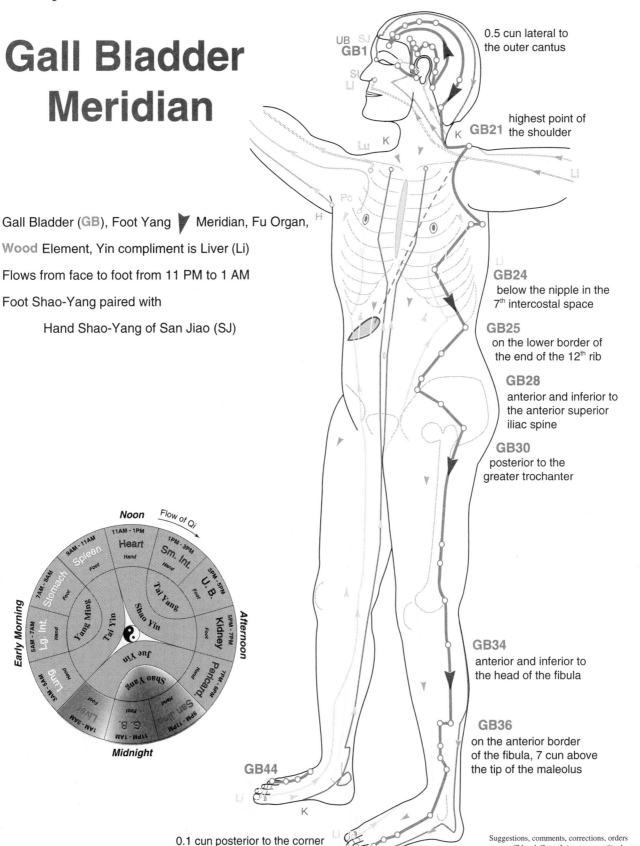

0.5 cun lateral to the outer cantus

GB21 highest point of the shoulder

GB24 below the nipple in the 7th intercostal space

GB25 on the lower border of the end of the 12th rib

GB28 anterior and inferior to the anterior superior iliac spine

GB30 posterior to the greater trochanter

GB34 anterior and inferior to the head of the fibula

GB36 on the anterior border of the fibula, 7 cun above the tip of the maleolus

GB44

0.1 cun posterior to the corner of the nail of the 4th toe

GB44

Suggestions, comments, corrections, orders contact Zdenek Zumr LAc. at zzumr@aol.com; Gall Bladder Meridian © Z. Zumr 2003

Gall Bladder: Also called a "Curious" organ.
- Holds and releases bile.
- Aids digestion, proper function helps extraction of "pure Substances".
- Its close tie with the Liver make it susceptible to upset from emotional stagnation.
- Rules decision-making.

Graphic: Zang/Fu Syndromes: Gall Bladder

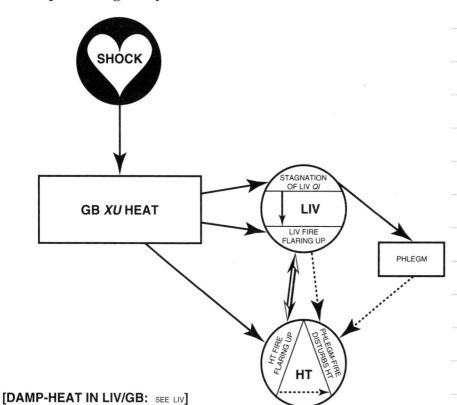

[DAMP-HEAT IN LIV/GB: SEE LIV**]**

Graphic: Liver Meridian

Liver Meridian

Liver (LI), Foot Yin ⬆ Meridian, Zang Organ,

Wood Element, Yang compliment is Gall Bladder (GB)

Flows from foot to chest from 1 AM to 3 AM

Foot Jue-Yin paired with
Hand Jue-Yin of Pericardium (Pc)

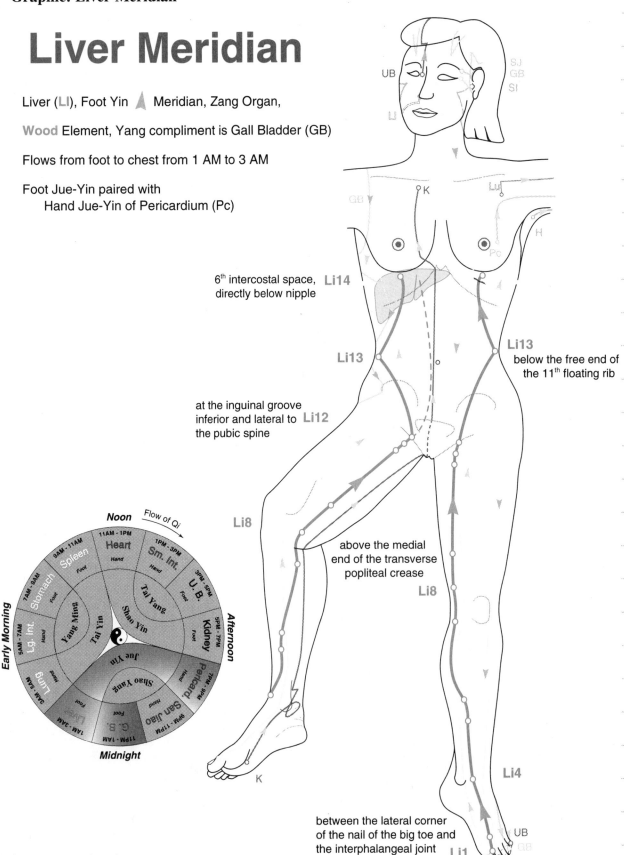

6th intercostal space,
directly below nipple — Li14

Li13

Li13
below the free end of
the 11th floating rib

at the inguinal groove
inferior and lateral to — Li12
the pubic spine

Li8

above the medial
end of the transverse
popliteal crease

Li8

Li4

between the lateral corner
of the nail of the big toe and
the interphalangeal joint
Li1

Suggestions, comments, corrections, orders contact
Zdenek Zumr LAc. at zzumr@aol.com; Liver Meridian © Z. Zumr 2003

Liver: Smooth movement of Qi & Xue, emotions
- "Free and easy wanderer" versus feeling stuck
- Expression, and flow of emotions
- See with open eyes, colors versus black&white, tunnel vision
- Control of emotions → depression, aggression

Graphic: Zang/Fu Syndromes: Liver

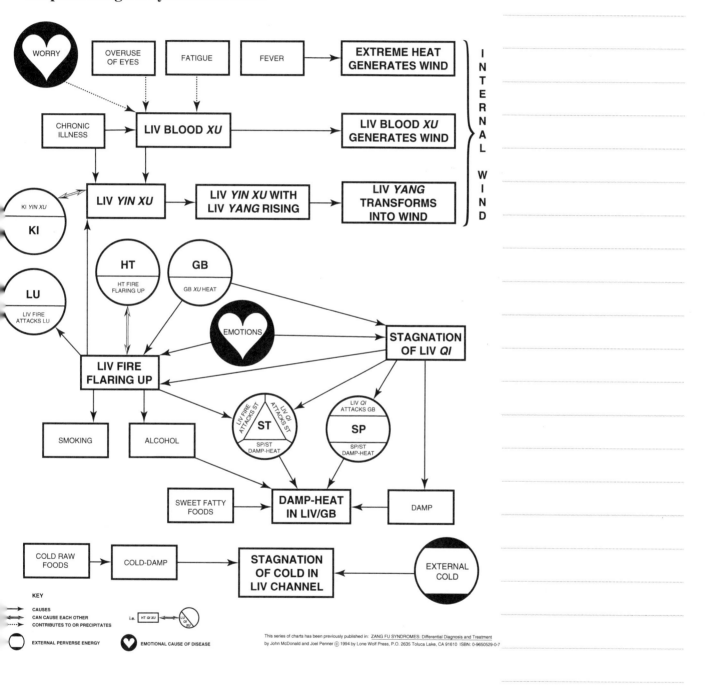

This series of charts has been previously published in: ZANG FU SYNDROMES: Differential Diagnosis and Treatment
by John McDonald and Joel Penner © 1994 by Lone Wolf Press, P.O. 2635 Toluca Lake, CA 91610 ISBN: 0-9650529-0-7

Eight Extra Meridians
Ren/Du, Conception and Governing Vessels

Chinese medicine has 12 organ meridians that are associated with internal organs. These 12 meridians are defined by their own points. Additionally there are 8 extra meridians. These meridians have balancing functions in the body and they are not associated with internal organs. Of those Eight Extra meridians only two have their own points:

- **Ren, aka. Conception Vessel** (Yin)
- **Du, aka. Governing Vessel** (Yang)

The Du channel is responsible for collecting and redistributing all Yang in the body and for bringing Yang Qi to the head. It runs from posterior to the anus, across the spine, over the midline of the head and face to terminate between the upper jaw and upper lip inside the mouth.

The Ren channel is responsible for collecting and redistributing all Yin in the body. It runs from anterior to the anus, across the genitalia, up the midline in front of the body to terminate below the lower lip.

The Ren and Du channels circumnavigate the digestive tract.

The other six of the Eight Extras don't have points of their own. They are defined by points from the 12 organ meridians. Consult reference material on the subject.*

There are a number of connecting paths and branches that connect the meridians to their respective organs, that connect Yin/Yang paired vessels, that connect the meridians to the Ren and Du channels and that serve extraordinary functions. These branches don't have names or points. They are not accessible for treatment and serve mostly to tie together TCM theory.

- Thus the question: "How many channels are there in Chinese medicine?" Answer → 20 Channels.
- Thus the question: "How many organ channels are there in Chinese medicine?" Answer → 12 Channels.
- Thus the question: "How many channels have their own points?" Answer → 14 Channels.

*These are the other six Extra meridians:
Yin Qiao/Yang Qiao (Yin Heel/Yang Heel)
Yin Wei/Yang Wei (Yin Linking/Yang Linking)
Chong and Dai (Penetrating/Girdle Vessel)

Graphic: Ren Meridian

Ren (Conception Vessel)
Yin Meridian

Yang compliment is Du
(aka. Governing Vessel)

The Ren Meridian is one of the Eight Extra Meridians
and thus not associated with an organ, rather it serves
to balance all Yin meridians in the body.

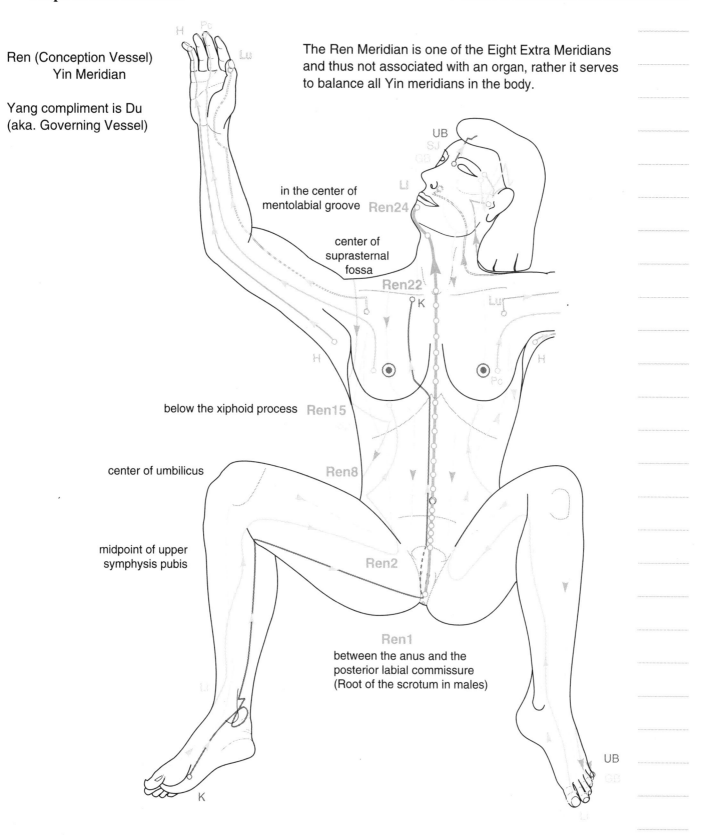

in the center of
mentolabial groove

Ren24

center of
suprasternal
fossa

Ren22

below the xiphoid process   Ren15

center of umbilicus   Ren8

midpoint of upper
symphysis pubis

Ren2

Ren1
between the anus and the
posterior labial commissure
(Root of the scrotum in males)

Graphic: Du Meridian

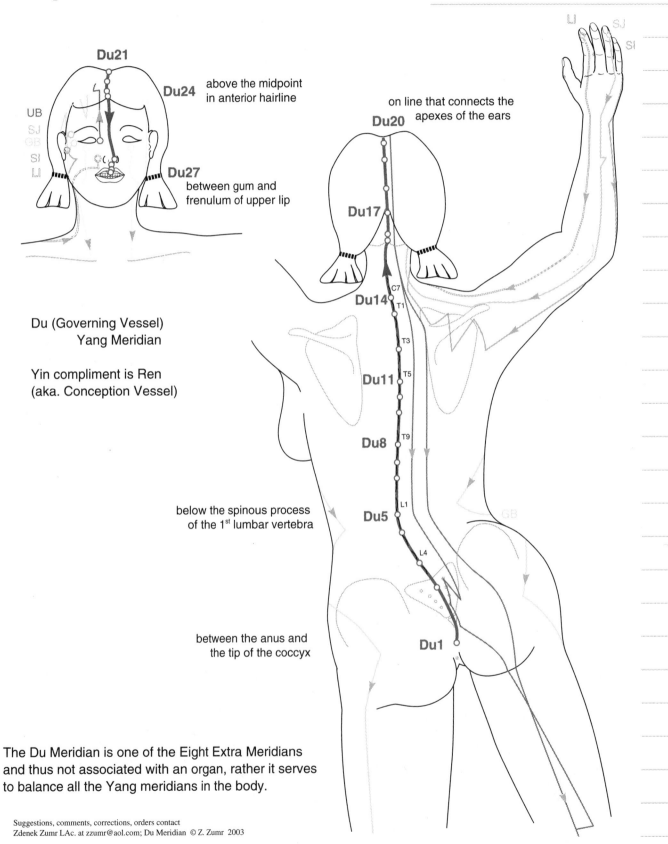

Du21

Du24
above the midpoint
in anterior hairline

Du27
between gum and
frenulum of upper lip

UB
SJ
GB
SI
LI

Du (Governing Vessel)
Yang Meridian

Yin compliment is Ren
(aka. Conception Vessel)

below the spinous process
of the 1st lumbar vertebra

between the anus and
the tip of the coccyx

on line that connects the
apexes of the ears

Du20

Du17

Du14 C7 / T1

T3

Du11 T5

Du8 T9

Du5 L1

L4

Du1

LI SJ
SI

GB

The Du Meridian is one of the Eight Extra Meridians
and thus not associated with an organ, rather it serves
to balance all the Yang meridians in the body.

Suggestions, comments, corrections, orders contact
Zdenek Zumr LAc. at zzumr@aol.com; Du Meridian © Z. Zumr 2003

Notes

Pathogenesis
If Qi flows strongly and smoothly, emotions are in balance, defenses are strong, spirits are high optimal health will result. If either of these factors become disturbed the defensive Qi will weaken and pathogens may enter the body or internal pathologies may arise.

Internal Pathologies
All emotions are healthy and normal unless experienced in excess or avoided or held over a long period of time, these are the pathologies that may result from such excess.

Graphic: Seven Emotions

Joy — scatters Qi, loss of focus, affects the Heart

  Pensiveness — ties up the Qi, brooding, obsessing, damages the Spleen

 Sadness — dissolves Qi, robs body of Qi, separation, release, affects the Lung

Grief — chronic excessive sadness, affects the Lung and Heart

Fear — descends Qi, damages the Kidneys or is caused by Kidney Qi deficiency (aging)

Fright — sudden descend of Qi, loss of control, panic, hit to the Kidney but also Heart

Anger — makes Qi rise, moodiness, repressed anger, depression, affects or is caused by Liver

Pathologies of Qi
- **Qi stagnation** – smooth flow is interrupted → pains and aches that move in the body
- **Qi Deficiency** – not enough Qi produced → tired, worn out easily, poor sleep, poor digestion
- **Sinking of Qi** – Qi descending → spirit is down, feeling heavy, can't smile
- **Qi Disharmony/Rebellious Qi** – Qi is not moving where it is supposed to → vomiting, head aches, tremors.

Six External Pathogens

With a strong Qi one can resist these pathogens longer or alleviate them faster. A conscious lifestyle can prevent these pathogens from arising altogether.

*   **Wind** – weather change, or a draft that enters the body creating wandering aches and pain
*   **Heat** – overheating on a hot day, dehydration, heat stroke
*   **Cold** – lowered body temperature, colds
*   **Dampness** – over eating, too much ice cream, salads, fruits
*   **Dryness** – not enough fluid intake, dry eyes, skin, dry mucus membranes, cracked lips
*   **Summer heat** – heat and dampness combined, hot spicy foods, too much alcohol

Other Factors

Diet

Proper food intake will guarantee plentiful generation of Qi. Improper food intake will inhibit generation of Qi and can introduce pathogens to the body that damage Spleen/Stomach thus preventing Qi generation.

*   **Overeating is #1 pathology**, particularly with cravings for fat or sugar
*   Intake of raw, cold or processed food
*   Eating spicy, hot, fried foods with alcohol
*   Phlegm disease, retention/generation of phlegm due to intake of foods that one can not digest; milk in most people

Lifestyle

Overwork: Using Qi faster than it is generated.

*   Physical overworking will impact on the Kidneys
*   Mental overwork will damage the Spleen
*   Emotional overwork will drain the Heart

Sex: Depletes Kidneys and Jing but that depletion can be made up unless:

*   when sick or tired (overworked)
*   when practiced when ill
*   poor hygiene
*   in excess
*   at a too young age
*   under the influence of drugs
*   during menstruation

Stress: Depletes Kidneys, distracts from what is really important.

Trauma

Accidents do happen! Even to good people. When accidents happen in a pattern investigate root cause.

*   Bodily injuries, surgery, broken bones
*   Any kind of injury due to parasites, insect bites, exposure to toxins
*   Unpredictable events, emotional distress, death in family

Wrong Treatment

*   Conditions that are misdiagnosed and treated which then result in more severe conditions
*   Aggravation of latent pathologies
*   Progressions from mild to severe
*   Use of wrong herbs for a given condition or abuse of herbal formulae (herbal weight loss trough Ma Huang, Coffee, Guarana, ...)

Notes

Diagnosis

There are several ways to diagnose in TCM. The practitioner choice depends on the pathology at hand, or which school of thought is employed. Diagnosis can utilize the Five Elements imbalances, meridian dysfunction, Organ (Zang/Fu) problems, Yin/Yang disharmony, patologies of Qi, etc.

One of the methods is to lay out the pathology according to the Eight Differentiations to clarify the treatment approach.

Graphic: Eight Differentiations

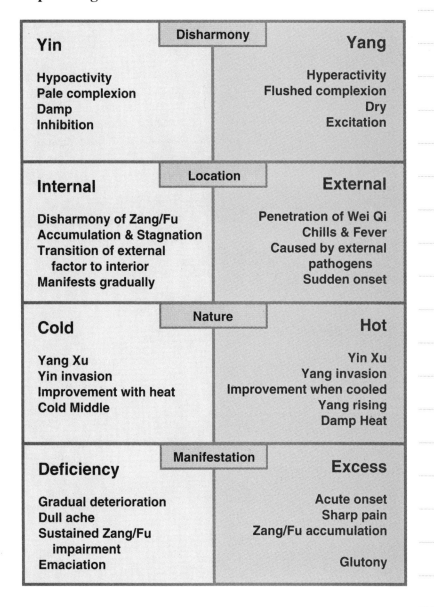

Disharmony	
Yin	**Yang**
Hypoactivity	Hyperactivity
Pale complexion	Flushed complexion
Damp	Dry
Inhibition	Excitation

Location	
Internal	**External**
Disharmony of Zang/Fu	Penetration of Wei Qi
Accumulation & Stagnation	Chills & Fever
Transition of external	Caused by external
factor to interior	pathogens
Manifests gradually	Sudden onset

Nature	
Cold	**Hot**
Yang Xu	Yin Xu
Yin invasion	Yang invasion
Improvement with heat	Improvement when cooled
Cold Middle	Yang rising
	Damp Heat

Manifestation	
Deficiency	**Excess**
Gradual deterioration	Acute onset
Dull ache	Sharp pain
Sustained Zang/Fu	Zang/Fu accumulation
impairment	
Emaciation	Glutony

Notes

Treatment Modalities

Chinese Medicine is the framework that allows for diagnosis. Acupuncture is one of several treatment modalities.

When treatment modalities are used outside the diagnosis methods, the proper selection of points is impossible and the disease is treated versus the patient. That approach is reminiscent of western style medicine.

BOUND & GAGGED

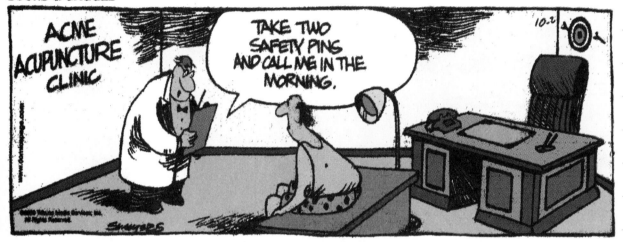

Acupuncture

After a thorough history and examination by a Chinese medicine practitioner a diagnosis is made in terms of Qi, Xue, Yin, Yang, 5 Elements, etc.

Appropriate points are selected and needles inserted. Insertion can be perpendicular or at angles, with or against the flow in the channel, stimulated to sedate or tonify, superficial or deep, left in for a while or just a skin prick depending on the intent of the practitioner. The overall condition is of importance as well as relative strength of pathology.

Needles range from 1.5 mm ($1/_{16}$") to 150 mm (6") in length and 0.12 mm to 0.35 mm in diameter. They are typically solid stainless steel needles with one end wrapped with copper wire or with an injection molded plastic handle. Stainless steel needles are always disposable.

Needles can also be made from silver, gold or other metals for a desired therapeutic effect. These are specialty needles and would be purchased by the patient and used only by this patient. In between treatments they would be cleaned and autoclaved.

Electro-Acupuncture

This is acupuncture with mild to intense stimulation by means of pulsating electrical currents. Great treatment of tight muscles and painful sports injuries.

Acupuncture Facials

Diminish the appearance of wrinkles, crows feet and frown lines without toxins. Treatments take only 15 minutes and the effects last for several hours up to several days.

Moxa

Is the fury undercoat of the Mugwort leaf that is scraped from the leaf, collected and then compressed into various forms. It can be placed directly on acupuncture points, wrapped around the shaft of a needle after it has been inserted or placed in a dish and burned. In either case it will glow and produce a heating sensation. In a cigar shaped form it can be burned 1-2" above the abdomen to warm up the area; the goal is to let the heat penetrate deeply thus it can relieve menstrual cramping. Moxa can also be filled into eye pillows to relax tired eyes, it can be placed in neck rolls to induce sleep.

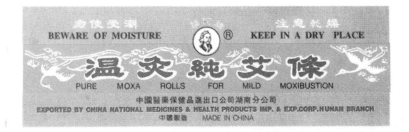

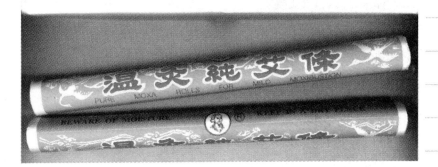

Mineral Lamps
Also called TDP Lamp. This is a therapeutic infrared (heating) device from China. The TDP has a plate coated with a mineral formulation including 33 elements derived from special clay. When heated the plate emits electromagnetic energy in the infrared range, which coincide with the bio-spectrum of the human body. The TDP lamp has proven to be effective in the relief of pains and in treating chronic ailments like; Arthritis, soft tissue, bone injuries, lumbago, wounds, carpel tunnel, disk problems, skin conditions. Each treatment lasts about 20 to 60 minutes.

Consultations
Everything you always wanted to know about TCM and never knew whom to ask. Demystifying preconceived notions about oriental medicine can open the door for patients with illnesses that defy western medical treatment.

Manual Techniques
Shiatsu
Originated in Japan. In this form of massage, pressure is applied with thumbs in small circular, or in short linear motions, followed by deep penetrating pressure to points, in a pattern that conforms to meridians from Chinese Medical Theory. While the pressure on individual points is reminiscent of Acupressure or trigger points therapy, the emphasis is on moving the flow of Qi in the body. A Shiatsu treatment usually includes the entire body or one whole side of the body.

Since the movements are very localized Shiatsu can be performed on fully clothed people, making it suitable for short treatments, treatments in public, office or business settings, or for people who prefer to remain clothed due to religious, social or cultural restrictions.

The treatments aim to release muscle tensions, such as computer neck, relieve headaches, back pain, menstrual pain and induce relaxation.

JinShinDo

Utilizing thumb and finger pressure in various locations of the body to induce a therapeutic effect. Points are held longer and deeper than in Shiatsu. Slower and less invasive than Shiatsu.

Tui-Na

Chinese style manipulations consisting of stretches and musculo-skeletal adjustments, reminiscent of Chiropractic Treatments.

An-ma; Am-ma

Chinese style abdominal massage. Great for children, people with digestive problems or for menstrual discomfort. Improves digestion and loosens bowel movements.

Cupping

Pyrex glass or plastic cups of varying sizes are applied to the body by a vacuum. The vacuum is created either with a pump or by heating the air on the inside of the cups by burning an alcohol soaked gauze in them. The jars are applied to the body and suck in the skin to bring blood to the surface, and with it pathogens that cause a disruption of the smooth flow of Qi. The cups are left on the patient for a short time. Modification of the treatment can include pricking the skin or inserting a needle under the cup first.

GuaSha

Utilizing a porcelain spoon or similar object with smooth round edges the skin is scraped. This brings blood to the surface in the treated area.

Notes

Herbs

The Chinese herbal pharmacopia includes over 10,000 items that have been described as medicinally useful. It includes all parts of plants, minerals, metals, all kinds of animal parts and excretions, including some human parts. Many herbs have been analyzed and were found to contain antibacterial and anti-viral substances, while others don't seem to contain any chemical substances with discernible effects. Yet other herbs are considered toxic by western standards. It is important to use herbs in the context described in classical texts, since often, within the prescriptions herbs are used to neutralize toxicity, harmonize the effects of ingredients or reverse the action of another herb. Quantities are to be adhered to unless advised by trained Chinese medical pharmacists. Too little can have no effect while too much could invert the function of an herb or cause toxicity. There are forbidden combinations and mutually enhancing effects that need to be taken into account when writing a prescription. Centuries of observation have made Chinese herbal remedies safe and effective to use but beware of fad products such as weight loss pills. There is no such thing as a TCM herbal weight loss formula.

Graphic: Pure, Herbal, Natural=Healthy?

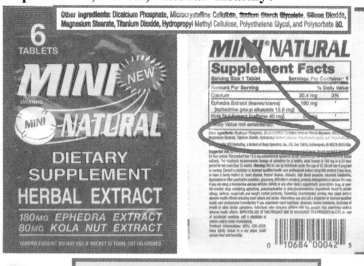

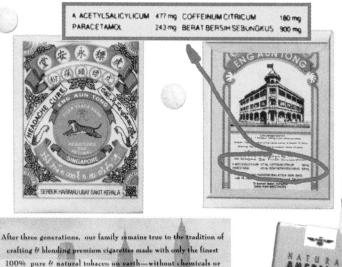

Diet

The most effective herbs is the food eaten every day. Eat with the seasons. Maintain a staple of different grains. How many do you know? Many pathologies arise from an unbalanced diet and can be resolved with dietary adjustments. The important part is to get a proper assessment first, so you know what to eat and when. If you want to loose weight broaden the variety of foods you eat - don't restrict. Most people maintain a too monotone diet where few items make up the bulk of caloric intake. Observe serving sizes and <u>never</u> eat at all-you-can-eat buffet.

Nutritional advise is easy to come by – every week there is a new miracle diet that promises to cure all ills, stop aging, and results in weight loss without effort or excercise. And then you grow up.

Before you fall for fad diets try to eat according to either of these tried and true food pyramids. Once you've mastered adherence to these pyramids you can start modifying them for your special needs and tastes.

Graphic: Western Food Pyramid

The Food Pyramid is based on recomendations for daily diatery intake.
Amounts of servings needs to be adjusted for activity levels and special needs.
If more calories are consumed then expended the excess will be retained as fat,
if fever calories are consumed then expended weight loss will result.

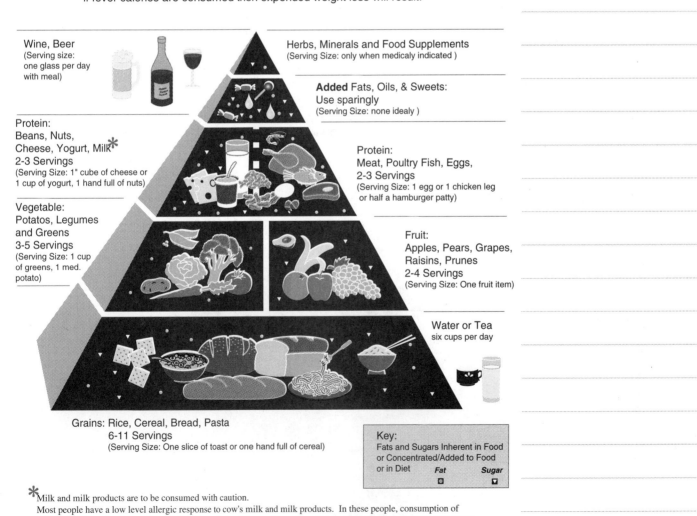

Wine, Beer
(Serving size:
one glass per day
with meal)

Herbs, Minerals and Food Supplements
(Serving Size: only when medicaly indicated)

Added Fats, Oils, & Sweets:
Use sparingly
(Serving Size: none idealy)

Protein:
Beans, Nuts,
Cheese, Yogurt, Milk*
2-3 Servings
(Serving Size: 1" cube of cheese or
1 cup of yogurt, 1 hand full of nuts)

Protein:
Meat, Poultry Fish, Eggs,
2-3 Servings
(Serving Size: 1 egg or 1 chicken leg
or half a hamburger patty)

Vegetable:
Potatos, Legumes
and Greens
3-5 Servings
(Serving Size: 1 cup
of greens, 1 med.
potato)

Fruit:
Apples, Pears, Grapes,
Raisins, Prunes
2-4 Servings
(Serving Size: One fruit item)

Water or Tea
six cups per day

Grains: Rice, Cereal, Bread, Pasta
6-11 Servings
(Serving Size: One slice of toast or one hand full of cereal)

Key:
Fats and Sugars Inherent in Food
or Concentrated/Added to Food
or in Diet   *Fat*   *Sugar*

*Milk and milk products are to be consumed with caution.
Most people have a low level allergic response to cow's milk and milk products. In these people, consumption of
milk and milk products as well as food aditives derived from milk such as whey, casein, and lactoglobulin will create
a variety of symptoms that will depend on the constitution of an individual. For more information look up:

http://www.farrp.org/articles/dairyfree.htm
http://www.ama-assn.org/ama/pub/category/8753.html#3

Graphic: TCM Food Pyramid

Rather then specify a daily dietary intake the TCM Food Pyramid is
balanced over the period of a month. Emphasis is on variety over quantity.

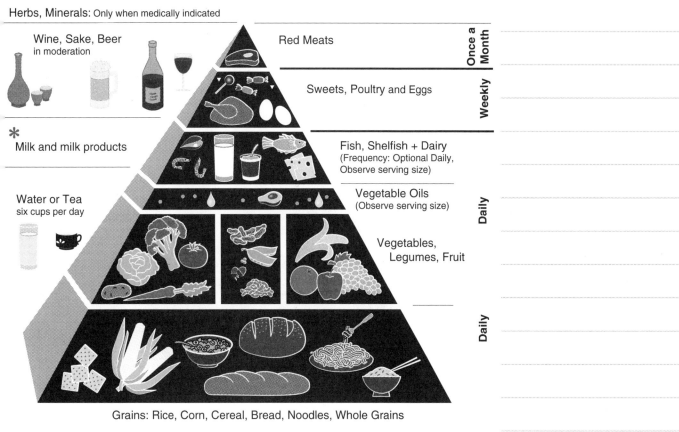

Grains: Rice, Corn, Cereal, Bread, Noodles, Whole Grains

* Milk and milk products are to be consumed with caution.
In TCM, milk creates phlegm that impedes the propper function of the digestive system and inhibits
the flow of Qi. Most people have a low level allergic response to cow's milk and milk products.
In these people, consumption of milk and related products will create a variety of symptoms that will
depend on the constitution of the individual.

Serving Size: If you gain weight you eat too much
If you loose weight you're not eating enough

Key:
Fats and Sugars Inherent in Food
or Concentrated/Added to Food
or in Diet   Fat   Sugar

In TCM foods are assessed in terms ofr Yin/Yang, hot/cold and meals will be
balanced appropriatly to the season and climate.   All foods have
physiological/medicinal properties that can be utilized to prevent/treat minor
discomforts. Furthermore the food pyramid is perfected by food grade herbs
that are used in daily cooking. Theese herbs do not constitute medicinal
formulae but they can balance the inherent quilities of foods, make them
more digestable, aid in elimination or address special nutritional needs of an
individual.

A good cook can keep the doctor at bay.

Read: → <u>Healing with Whole Foods</u> by Paul Pitchford

Graphic: Vegetarian Food Pyramid

The Vegetarian Food Pyramid is balanced in every meal. Animal products are o.k. as long as the animal remains unharmed. Foods are combined to provide full nutritional support and for ease of digestion.

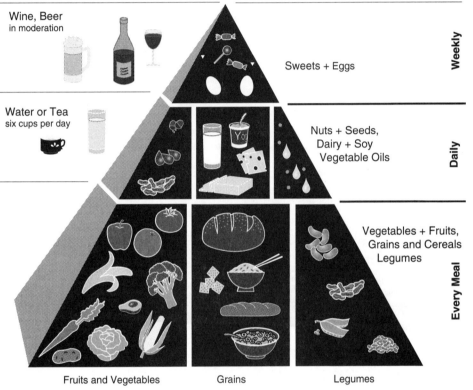

Herbs, Minerals: Only when medically indicated

Wine, Beer
in moderation

Water or Tea
six cups per day

Weekly

Sweets + Eggs

Daily

Nuts + Seeds,
Dairy + Soy
Vegetable Oils

Every Meal

Vegetables + Fruits,
Grains and Cereals
Legumes

Fruits and Vegetables   Grains   Legumes

Serving Size: If you gain weight you eat too much.
If you loose weight you're not eating enough.

Key:
Fats and Sugars Inherent in Food
         Fat   Sugar

Vegetarian traditions can be found in many cultures and revolve around the idea that to maintain one's spiritual integrity taking another beeings life should be avoided. Since it is perfectly possible to have a balanced and nutritious diet without having to kill animals for sustenance many choose this option.

Arguments have been made as to the health, nutritional, environmental, social, political benefits of vegeterianism. To evaluate the relevance of these arguments remains the responsibility of the individual.

Spiritual Practices

Maintain some practice that allows you to change perspectives on your existence.

- **Embrace**: Rituals, religious practices, groups that welcome anyone.
- **Beware**: Of those that ask for money to show you the way.
- **Run**: From those that build their following on claims of superiority or the exclusion of others.

Self-cultivation: You are the creator of your universe; the better the architect, the better the creation.

Be humble, remember the universe doesn't revolve around you.

Lifestyle

Live now. Don't wait until you have money to have a good time.
Spend money on self improvement not on things.
Many pathologies arise from an unhealthy life style. To much of a good
thing is as damaging as too much of a bad thing. Anything in excess will
damage the Qi → Too much food, drugs, sex, fear, joy, money.

Follow the Healing Pyramid to leave behind detrimental practices, move up
in self-cultivation.

Graphic: Healing Pyramid

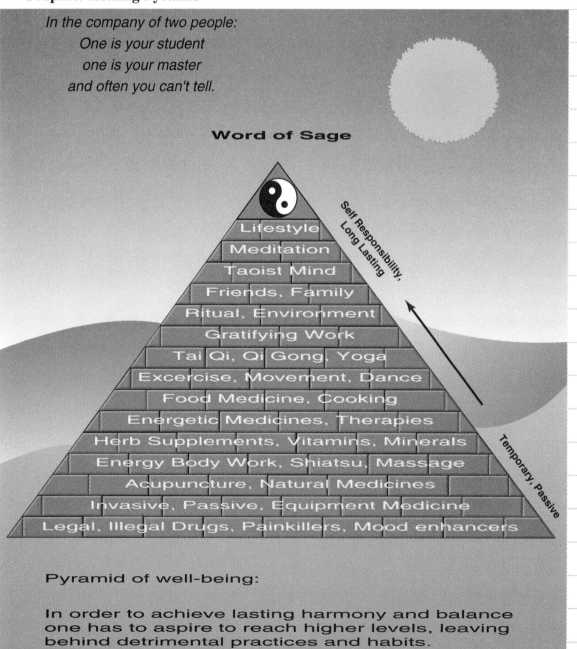

In the company of two people:
   One is your student
   one is your master
and often you can't tell.

Word of Sage

Self Responsibility, Long Lasting

Lifestyle
Meditation
Taoist Mind
Friends, Family
Ritual, Environment
Gratifying Work
Tai Qi, Qi Gong, Yoga
Excercise, Movement, Dance
Food Medicine, Cooking
Energetic Medicines, Therapies
Herb Supplements, Vitamins, Minerals
Energy Body Work, Shiatsu, Massage
Acupuncture, Natural Medicines
Invasive, Passive, Equipment Medicine
Legal, Illegal Drugs, Painkillers, Mood enhancers

Temporary, Passive

Pyramid of well-being:

**In order to achieve lasting harmony and balance
one has to aspire to reach higher levels, leaving
behind detrimental practices and habits.
Each higher level represents greater self
reliance and well-being.**

Valuable point selections for the massage therapist

These points have a generally recognized and somewhat singular function. Of course nothing replaces proper diagnosis but these points lend themselves to simple generalizations.

The points can be stimulated by, or Moxa can be burned and the points warmed. All points exist bilateral, so that if the intended point is not accessible or contraindicated due to its location, use the opposite site.

Use common sense! No point should cause more pain in treatment than is present with the pathology.

4 Gates for Qi stagnation.
Large Intestine 4 and Liver 3, "4 Gates", between the thumb and the index finger; between the big toe and adjacent toe, one thumb width above the junction. For feeling stuck, depression, agitation, unspecified moving aches and pain.

Stomach 25, Ren12, Ren 6, "4 Doors".
Points two finger breath, below and to either side and a hand width above the umbilicus and a hand width above. For constipation, diarrhea, bloating, belching, etc.

Gall Bladder 21, GB 21 for ascending Yang.
Highest point of shoulder, grab the muscle and pinch it. For many types of headache, tight shoulders, "too many thoughts in the head", restlessness, temper, etc.

Stomach 36, St 36 great point to increase overall energy in body.
One hand width below the lateral condyle of the tibia, two finger breath lateral to the tibia. Preferably treat with Moxa, do not use with external disease progress. For tiredness, weak digestion, feeling cold, etc.

Spleen 6, Sp 6 great point to increase overall energy in body, especially for women and menstrual problems. One hand width above the medial malleolus one finger breath posterior to the bone. Preferably treat with Moxa, do not use with external disease progress. For tiredness, weak digestion, feeling cold, etc.

Gall Bladder 34, GB 34 great point for the tendons.
Directly below the lateral condyle of the tibia. In most people this is a tender spot. To increase flexibility on the tendons and any kind of tendonitis, massage this point until soft.

Urinary Bladder 10, UB 10 or An Mian relax, induce sleep.
At the base of the occiput, 1-3 finger breath away from the midline.
Gently massage the area or place head on a neck roll.

Heart 7, 6, 5, H7, 6, 5 calm the heart.
On the ulnar side, about 1-2 finger breath above the wrist crease.
Gently rub the area or grab you fore arm along the Ulna.

Notes

Notes

Notes

Ayurvedic medicine

This type of medicine is practiced mostly on the Indian subcontinent. Although some of the concepts may seem similar to the Chinese medicine model, the two should not be mixed.

Ayurveda raises the claim that it is the oldest system of health care in continuous practice in the world.

Ayuh – means life
Veda – means knowledge or study
Thus combined *Ayurveda* means "the study of life" or "study of life-span"

* Deals with mind body and spirit.
* Includes herbs, diet, exercises (various forms of Yoga), and hands-on techniques.
* Geared towards prevention, and treatment of root cause, not suppression of symptoms.
* Stresses individual approach to well being as well as self-care.
* Recognizes physiological, psychological and emotional causes of disease.
* Health is the result of a harmony between mind body and soul, the body can not be cured without a healthy mind and healthy soul
* Stresses balance within the Five Elements and harmony between ones archetype and lifestyle

Stresses importance of proper diet and good digestion to provide protection from pathologies.

Unlike TCM that experienced a great unification of a variety of styles and schools of thought in the 1950's, Ayurvedic medicine continues to evolve along many paths. Through reduction, TCM created a foundation that was extracted from traditional practices that now can easily be communicated in a classroom setting. This reduction involved the elimination of religious and spiritual references as well as the elimination of mysticism. In Ayurvedic medicine these elements are included and, depending on the school of thought, may dominate the practice approach. As with many religious and mystical practices, information between sources may be vague, conflicting or even contradictory.

In this approach I try to communicate key concepts of Ayurveda that are uniformly recognized.

The practice of Aura and Chakra readings and treatments is one that exists separately from Ayurvedic medicine but is often practiced in conjunction.

Five Elements

At the base of this medical system lie Five Elements that represent inherent qualities of objects or processes. It is important to note that the relationship governing these Five Elements is one of evolution rather then interaction. These are not the same Five Elements that exist in Chinese medicine.

Graphic: Ayurvedic Five Elements

ETHER: Etheric forms of matter, space infinity, interconnectedness

Location, tissues
Head, mind, senses

Qualities, "Gunas"
cold, dry, without form, smooth

AIR: Gaseous form, subtle movement

Location, tissues
Nose, chest, respiration, circulation

Qualities, "Gunas"
cold, dry, light, smooth

FIRE: Heat, radiation, light

Location, tissues
Abdomen, digestive tract, small intestine

Qualities, "Gunas"
hot, dry, light active, smooth

WATER: Water, liquids, flowing movement

Location, tissues
Lower abdomen, uro-genital tract, reproductive organs

Qualities, "Gunas"
cold, wet, heavy active, smooth

EARTH: Solid, stable, resisting

Location, tissues
Anus, appendages

Qualities, "Gunas"
cold, dry, heavy solid, rough

(Left axis, top to bottom: Less Dense → More Dense; Trough Power of Transformation; arrows labeled Movement, Friction, Thickening, Coagulation)

Note: These are not the same Five Elements from Chinese medicine introduced earlier in this text

Note that some of the qualities ascribed to the Elements are overlapping, thus necessitating consideration of all qualities to determine the nature of an object rather then selecting a singular aspect.

Doshas

Also referred to as the Tridosha System, or Humors they are:

Vata   –   (Air) moving process
Pita   –   (Fire) digestive process
Kapha   –   (Water and Earth) body

Ayurveda is based on careful analysis of these Doshas as they make up the body and are the primary factors behind subtle changes in physiological or psychological states.

Graphic: Doshas / Humors

VATA: Air within space

Root of Humors; breathing, effort, movement "wind"

ETHER + AIR → Elements combine

Primary location, tissues	Qualities, "Gunas"
Colon, thighs, hips, ears, bones, musculo skeletal system	cold, dry, light, agitaded, rough

PITA: Fire contained by water

Digestive fire, power of transformation "bile"

FIRE + WATER → Elements combine

Location, tissues	Qualities, "Gunas"
Small Intestine, stomach, blood, sweat glands	hot, oily, penetrating, mobile, liquid

KAPHA: Water controlled by earth

Physical shape, holding together, adhesion "phlegm"

WATER + EARTH → Elements combine

Location, tissues	Qualities, "Gunas"
Stomach, chest, throat, head, pancreas, lymph, fat, tongue	cold, wet, heavy, slow, firm

These humors are not material, they are *not a sum* of the Elements that form them, rather they are *formed by the interaction* of the Elements.
In interacting with one another the Doshas account for:

• Creating and maintaining the body
• Perception and expression of emotions
• Pathologies

Other qualities associated with the archetypes:

DOSHAS	VATA	PITA	KAPHA
Formed by Elements	((Ether and) Air)	(Fire (and Water))	(Water and Earth)
Qualities	mobile dry cold subtle	mobile liquid hot penetrating	firm wet cold dull
Organs Tissues Senses	Nervous system thighs, hips, ear, bones, Touch	Liver stomach, sweat, sebaceous glands, blood, lymph, ... Vision	Plasma pancreas, connective tissue, fat, throat, ... Thought
Resides in: Time of Day	Colon 3PM - 7PM 3AM - 7AM	Small Intestine 11PM - 3AM 11AM - 3PM	Stomach 7PM - 11PM 7AM - 11AM
Development Life Stage	decline older than 50 (65)	manifestation adult 15 - 50 y/old	development childhood conception - 15 y/old
Life Style Live Life Excess Climate	irregular sleeping and eating ungrounded, unrealistic cold, dry, windy, high altitude, SW desert	regular sleeping and eating anger aggression hot, damp, tropical, middle elevation, east Texas	heavy sleeper overly dependent, dull, passive cold, damp, sea level, NW / New England
Personality Body type	Enthusiastic, bright, impulsive, moody Thin wiry	Quick, intelligent, predictable muscular, good build but can gain weight	Love, peace, comfort, stubborn, hateful, conflict solid, heavy

This list is by no means complete. Anything can be analyzed in relation to Doshas and more extensive lists can be found for foods, activities, life cycles etc. Bringing ones Archetype and lifecycle in harmony with the Tridosha system is a prescription for health and wealth in Ayurvedic medicine.

Vata
- Also called the Primary Humor
- Responsible for all physical processes and bodily functioning
- Governs movement, energy, breathing,
- Expresses emotional responses such as fear, anxiety, nervousness
- Enables intellectual flexibility and reasoning
- Source of Prana, "Life Force" that is derived mostly from breath, similar in concept to Chinese Qi

Essences - avoid florals
use warming stimulating oils: Clove, Cinnamon, Melissa
Base oils: Sesame, Hazelnut

Pita

- Responsible for all metabolic and chemical transformations, body heat
- Governs digestion, complexion
- Expresses hunger, thirst, intelligence, understanding; expresses in the eyes
- Enables perception of reality and intellectual understanding of reality
- Source of emotions of anger and hate

Essences: Champa, Jasmine, Rose, Violet, Mimosa
Base oils: Olive, Sunflower

Kapha

- Responsible for lubrication of joints and membranes
- Governs physical body that provides a home for other humors
- Expresses emotional states of sympathy and calm
- Enables the other Doshas to function in the body
- Source of emotions of love, attachment, greed, emotional understanding

Essences: Rosemary, Sage, Pine, Basil, Ginger, Black Pepper
Base oils: Almond, Apricot, Flaxseed

Graphic: 24 Hour Doshas

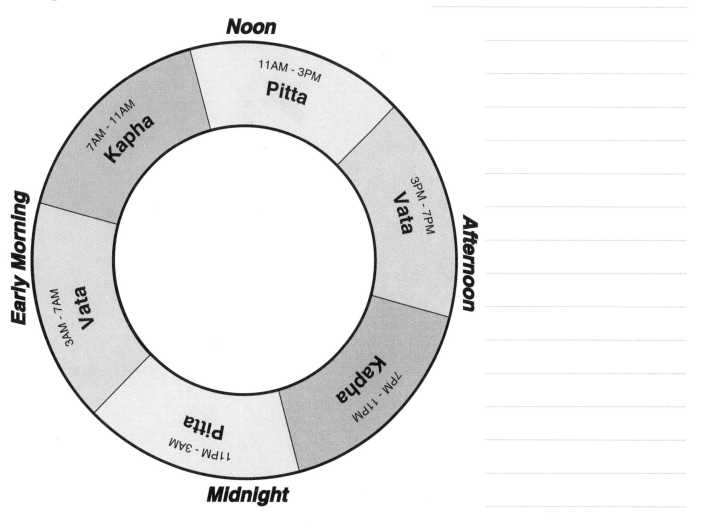

Archetypes / Constitutions

Determined at birth, can not be changed
Unique to each individual as a mixture of Doshas / Humors:

- None is better than the next; balance between the Doshas is key to health
- Know your constitution, as it will point to tendencies to pathological that, when recognized early will be easily corrected
- Constitution will govern individual response to pathological conditions
- Include both psychological and physiological body (Prakriti)
- Evolve lifestyle that supports constitutions
- Maintaining diet can support constitution
- Expression of constitution is highly individual, i.e. same basic constitutions can manifest differently
- Will determine treatment approach when pathologies are present

Graphic: Seven Archetypes

Singular

Double

Triple

VATA

Personality / Body type
Enthusiastic, bright, impulsive, moody / thin wiry body
Life style / excess
Irregular sleeping + eating / ungrounded, dreamer

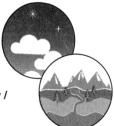

PITA

Personality / Body type
Quick, intelligent, predictable / muscular, good build
Life style / excess
regular sleeping eating / anger, argression

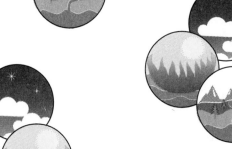

Double / Triple
Since there are positive and negative attributes ascribed to the Doshas as well as excesses and deficiencies, it is not necessarily an advantage to be of Dual or Triple Archetype.
Life style
The importance lies in fostering an awareness of, and conducting a lifestyle appropriate to one's archetype.

KAPHA

Personality / Body type
Loving, peaceful, comfortable, stubborn / solid, heavy
Life style / excess
heavy sleeper, gourmand / dependent, dull, passive

Seven Archetypes / Constitutions
- **Pure/Single**

Vata – (Air) moving process
Pita – (Fire) digestive process
Kapha – (Water and Earth) body

- **Dual**

Vata – Pita / (Air) moving process – (Fire) digestive process
Pita – Kapha / (Fire) digestive process – (Water and Earth) body
Kapha – Vata / (Water and Earth) body – (Air) moving process

- **Triple**

Vata – Pita – Kapha
(Air) moving process – (Fire) digestive process – (Water and Earth) body

The Archetypes are descriptive not determinative. Any of the seven archetypes offers qualities that when observed will lead to health and wealth, each of the seven archetypes also includes liabilities that when avoided will be of no consequence.

The Dual and Triple archetypes offer greater flexibility in one's personal expression. That flexibility may also be detrimental because it also includes susceptibility to more pathogens.

Pathogenesis

Pathogenesis revolves around the digestive function. If digestion is well plenty of **Prana** is present for daily activity as well as emotional stability. This digestive function is called **Agni**.

Prana is the Ayurvedic equivalent of life force, similar to the Chinese medicine concept of Qi.

- If Agni is balanced food will be digested completely, leaving no residue, creating a clear mind, awareness of the senses and pure spirit and emotions as well as an energetic body.

- If Agni is either, irregular, deficient or high, food will not be digested completely, leaving toxic residue that can accumulate and fester. This toxic mass can stagnate, ferment and cause disease. Symptoms will present as a dull mind, cloudy senses, skewed perception, confused spirit and heavy body and low immunity. Low immunity will give rise to all kinds of chronic ailments and susceptibility to pathogens.

Graphic: Progression of Disease

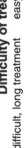

Difficulty of treatment:
easy, minor adjustments
difficult, long treatment

Accumulation:

Pathology
Humors accumulate in their respective locations

Treatment
Compensation, aromatic herbs,
easy to correct with early treatment

Aggravation:

Pathology
Continued accumulation manifests with symptoms outside of Humors

Treatment
Dispersion, cleansing herbs, fasting

Overflow:

Pathology
Humors fill up and overflow

Treatment
Reduction, give up excess

Migration:

Pathology
Overflow moves into tissues

Treatment
Clear pathways of overflow: Cleanse Humors (central pathway)
guide overflow to blood (inner pathway)
guide overflow to intestine (outer pathway)

Manifestation:

Pathology
Symptoms manifest in tissues with overflow

Treatment
Assess symptoms, tissues and treat accordingly

Diversification:

Pathology
Symptoms manifest over entire body, identifiable Humors

Treatment
Treat symptoms and Humors

Maintaining Agni

- The overall balance of Doshas and emotions affects Balance of Agni.
- Learn to experience and distinguish appetite, hunger, satiation, thirst v/s cravings, desires, impulsive/compulsive eating.
- Eat regularly, clean, fresh food. → Any processed, pre–cooked, chemically altered food will impede Agni.
- Take time to eat. Focus on eating. → Stress, emotional disturbance will stagnate digestion.
- Eat small and slow meals.

It is a common misconception that refrigerators can be used to keep food "fresh".

In Chinese as well as in Ayurvedic medicine the term "fresh" is applied only to food that is consumed no later then three days after it has been harvested. Only then will the food yield its full potential of generating Qi or Prana. This necessitates a lifestyle that requires frequent trips to farmers markets and a diet that is in sync with the seasons.

Refrigeration is just another form of preservation just like freezing, drying, canning, curing, etc. Anytime food is preserved it looses some of its ability to generate Qi, although it may still be nutritious from a western medicine point of view.

OVEREATING is the #1 Pathology
Giving rise to obesity, heart problems, high blood pressure, diabetes etc.

- Eat only when hungry – don't snack between meals (excess fat).
- Drink only when thirsty – water or tea are best (no sugar/caffeine/ice).
- Eat small meals that comply with the food Pyramid (lots of grains).
- Combine foods appropriately (season, climate, types of foods).
- Eat appropriate foods for you constitutional type.
- Learn and use herbs in the kitchen they are medicine.

Treatment Approach

- "What we do every day makes us who we are".
- Establish Life-regimens to follow on a daily, weekly, monthly yearly and lifecycle base.
- Keep regimens as well as life simple.
- Treatment of pathologies deals primarily with balancing the Doshas, recognizing the underlying imbalances; secondarily with recognition of pathogens.

Sattvic life style
Purity of body, pure diet, proper exercises, personal hygiene.
Purity of thought, honesty, humility, truthfulness.
Purity of soul, compassion, non-violence, giving up ego.
Purity of lifestyle environment, livelihood, speech.
Devotion to the divine, spiritual practice, meditation, service.

Ayurvedic Remedies

- Diet and herbal remedies

Indian food tends to be much more flavorful than western foods. Spices and herbs used in the preparation of meals have medicinal properties and imbalances can resolved with an appropriate meal. Herbal preparations in Ayurvedic medicine can be very complex and involve many steps, where herbs may be ground, boiled, fermented, distilled, aged and processed through complex chemical reactions. Few of these remedies have been evaluated for interactions with western medicines. The remedies can be very potent and their herbal origin doesn't mean that they will be well tolerated or harmless.

With the proliferation of herbal supplements onto supermarket shelves it is easy to forget that they still are medicines and should only be taken after consultation with trained professionals.

- Oils and massage
- Life style most notable factor in maintaining health: stress, drugs, addictions, relationships, sex, ...
- Physical life: Environment, climate, seasons, eating, digestion, elimination.
- Spiritual life: Choose one that is right for you; may or may not include ritual, congregation, deity, meditation, etc.
- Yoga, practice of breathing and movement exercises to strengthen the body and clear the mind.

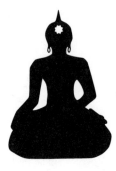

Notes

Notes

Auras and Chakras

The concept of Auras and Chakras is built on the idea that Prana (Life force) can be assessed by observing not only the physical body but also an "energetic" body. Rather than observing Prana itself its manifestations and pathologies can be perceived.

Aura is a byproduct of Prana and is formed by any living being. An Aura can have distinct qualities such as color, clarity, intensity, distribution, extension from the body, etc. The process of "seeing" Auras is highly individualistic and in the absence of a clear definition of what an Aura is remains unsubstantiated.

Chakras are also formed by the flow of Prana in the body. They are areas in which Prana gathers and becomes observable and treatable. There are seven major chakras and any number of additional minor chakras, namely in the hands, feet, genitalia, nape of the neck, along the spine, major joints etc. These chakras can be thought of as energy centers of the body where healthy Prana manifests (see associations page 100) or pathologies manifest if Prana is disturbed. Much like the Auric perceptions, the process of "seeing" or "feeling" Chakras is a highly individualistic one and in the absence of a clear definition of what Prana and therefore a Chakra is remains unproven.

However these systems are not without their merits. In popular language color perception in emotionally charged situations is well established and an accepted way of communicating impressions:

- A person who sees **red** is probably angry.
- A **yellowbelly** is somebody who shows cowardice.
- Feeling **blue** has built an entire genre of music devoted to melancholy.
- Ever seen a person that is **green** with envy?
- A person is also **green** when they are inexperienced.
- **White** represents innocence.
- Death and morbidity are seen as dark or **black**.

Depending on the culture these color perceptions may vary but they can be found around the world. Not everybody has the sensitivity to perceive emotions in fellow beings but that is a skill that can be trained through experience. Individuals that make it their profession to study people will acquire an acute awareness of a person's state of mind, motivation, fear, etc. simply by observing that persons appearance. That may include posture, facial expressions, complexion, mannerism, speech, voice, eye contact, physical contact, smell, and other less tangible qualities. When all impressions are considered a perception emerges. That perception may take the form of a color combination.

"**Seeing**" colors is a process that involves the physiology of the eyes and brain, a percentage of the population is color-blind, i.e. can not see colors. Colors that can be "seen" can be reproduced with photographic equipment.

"**Perceiving**" colors on the other hand, as defined above, is open to anybody including the blind since it involves all senses including the heart.

With this distinction the process of seeing Auras is no longer an esoteric gift to few, but rather a skill that anyone can acquire with experience and practice.

Auras

Auras offer a system by which to communicate and chart one's perceptions of an individuals state of mind.

Graphic: Radiating Auras

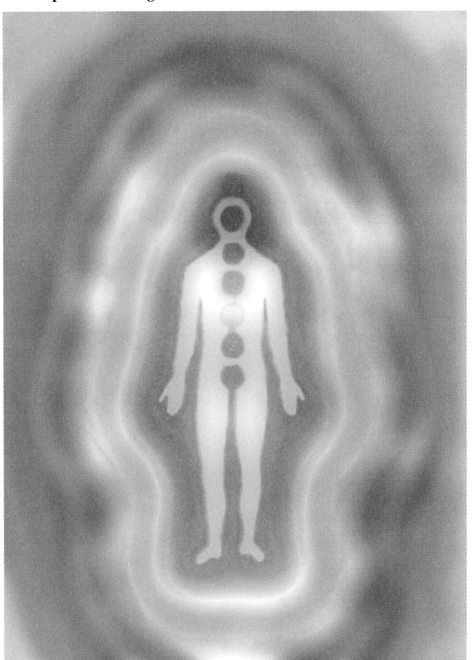

The aura is thought of as a continuous radiating field of infinite size that interconnects with all of creation, independent of distance and sometimes time. Interconnection means that one is affected by all auras and at the same time that one affects any and all auras independent of distance or intent.

For the purpose of instruction and clinical analysis the radiating field aura model is replaced with a more tangible layer model. In this model signs and symptoms of pathologies can be associated with individual aura layers that in turn can be manipulated trough various practices to elicit change and thus provide improvement in pathological conditions.

Graphic: Distinct Layers Aura

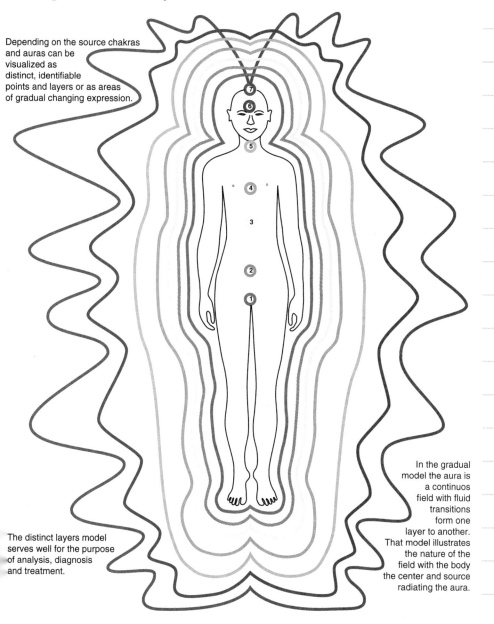

Depending on the source chakras and auras can be visualized as distinct, identifiable points and layers or as areas of gradual changing expression.

The distinct layers model serves well for the purpose of analysis, diagnosis and treatment.

In the gradual model the aura is a continuos field with fluid transitions form one layer to another. That model illustrates the nature of the field with the body the center and source radiating the aura.

To argue whether there is such a thing as a field that radiates into the outer reaches of the universe, or touches the hand of the divine is a moot point. What counts is an individual's perception of these entities that determines our assessment. If a patient presents with fear of the unknown, space aliens, the vengeful hand of god, it matters little to point out that there is no such thing. To the patient the fear is real and a treatment should be sought to alleviate that fear.

Listed are some of the factors that could be used to assess an individuals mental and spiritual health.

Outermost Purple Aura, associated with the 7th chakra:
Connection with all of creation, the universe and the divine. One is affected by anything that happens in the universe and beyond and vice versa., the idea of infinity in time and space.

6th Indigo Aura:
Connection to what is known, the visible universe, our solar system, planet Earth. → Astrology
The awareness that the way you conduct your life has an impact on every living thing on this planet, and anything that happens on this planet has an effect on you.

5th Blue Aura:
Connection with any living entity that you can communicate with in any way or that communicates with you. With the onset of the Internet that may be the entire planet but typically your community, family, acquaintances.
What you say will be heard; choose your expressions carefully.

4th Green Aura:
Connection with special individuals that at some point were or still are close to you; (long lost) friends, enemies, (ex-) lovers, (ex-) spouses, teachers, soul mates, masters, kindred spirits.

3rd Yellow Aura:
Connections with people that have an influence on you, whose opinion you value. Someone you get a "gut-feeling" about, worry about.

2nd Orange Aura:
Personal relationship, the one you want to be close to.
The one you want to procreate with. Somebody that invades your space and you don't mind.

1st Red Aura:
Connection with your Self. Know Thy Self.
What is it that you really want? Starts at the skin.

Pathologies are assessed by comparing "normal" or appropriate expressions with those present.
   Treatment modalities may involve colored lights, tones, sound frequencies, radio frequencies, gems, breathing or movement exercises, emotional, spiritual counseling and many more.
   Invariably the nature of a successful treatment is highly individual that may or may not be applicable generically.

Chakras

The earliest mention of chakras as psychic centers of consciousness in Yoga appears in the Upanishads (circa 600B.C.).   Three texts, the Gorakshashatakam and the Padaka-Pancaka, both written in the 10th century and the Sat-Cakra-Nirupana, written in 1577 contain descriptions of the centers and related practices as well as give instructions for meditating on the chakras. These texts form the foundation of chakras and Kundalini, which became an integral part of yoga philosophy.

The main text in the West about chakras was a translation by Arthur Avalon; The Serpent Power published in 1919.
    In these traditions, there are seven basic chakras, and they all exist within the subtle body, overlaying the physical body.

Chakra stands for the Sanscrit of "wheel". As such it implies movement and one should not think of the chakras as a static display but rather an ever-changing interplay of subtle energies.
    In Indian philosophy chakras are the expressions of consciousness, mental and spiritual forces that shape a person. Each chakra has associations to color, tone, sound, mantra, breath, the senses as well as spiritual and mental aspects.
    To be able to make informed decisions about oneself it is important that all chakras are in balance.
    From a western point of view the chakras have been equated with the endocrine system, the limbic system, the nervous system, instincts, intellectual pursuits, alchemistic symbols, etc.

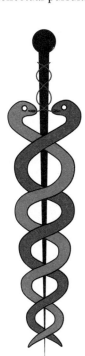

The chakras are interconnected with various pathways along which energies flow and can be balanced. There is a central channel that runs through the center of the spinal column and a pair of complementary channels, Ida (left) and Pingala (right) that express an interplay similar to Yin/Yang in TCM.
    Often the interplay is displayed as two snakes wrapped around a stake, not unlike the traditional logo of Western medicine.

There are many schools of thought and sources may disagree on many aspects. It is important not to perceive the chakra system as a factual explanation of the workings of the human mind/body but rather an artist interpretation or vision. Thus there is great variety in symbols, colors, associations.   Information may be sometimes overlapping, sometimes conflicting. Keep a flexible mind.

Chakra #1 Base

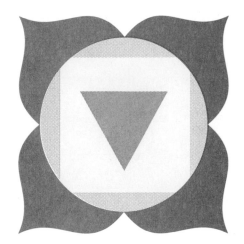

Located at the base of the spine, this chakra forms our foundation. It represents the element earth, and is therefore related to our survival instincts, and to our sense of grounding and connection to our bodies and the physical plane, physical identity, oriented to self-preservation.

This is the chakra that is connected to survival on the material plane.

When this chakra is disturbed one has fear about survival. When this chakra is balanced, one feels that one belongs on the earth, and is connected with its bounty health, prosperity, security, and dynamic presence.

Chakra #2, Sacral, Naval

The second chakra, located in the abdomen, lower back, and sexual organs, is related to the element water, and to emotions, emotional identity, oriented toward self-gratification and sexuality. It connects us to others through feeling, desire, sensation, and movement.

Balance in this chakra is manifested by balance and appropriateness in sexual activity, fluidity and grace, depth of feeling, sexual fulfillment, and the ability to accept changes by fertility (when appropriate) and creativity.

Chakra #3, Solar Plexus

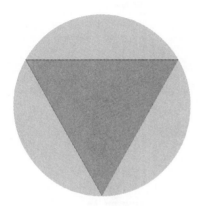

This chakra is the power chakra, located in the solar plexus, related to fire. It rules our personal power, will, ego identity, self-definition and autonomy, as well as our metabolism.

This is the chakra of digestion, energy, effectiveness, spontaneity, and non-dominating power. The ego can manifest itself for good or harm through the power of the navel chakra.

Chakra #4, Heart

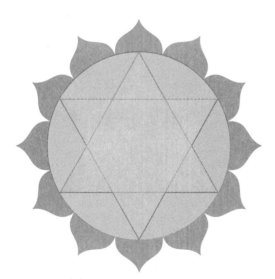

This chakra is the middle chakra in a system of seven; its element is air. It is related to love, self-acceptance and integrates complementary pairs such as: mind and body, male and female, ego and unity. A balanced fourth chakra allows us to love deeply, feel compassion, have a sense of peace and centeredness.

Balance in this chakra is expressed by empathy and caring for one self and others. This is represented by the shape of two triangles in the chakra, one pointing up, and the other down. This symbolizes being equally connected to the earth and heaven.

There is a shift at the level of the fourth chakra. While the first three chakras are associated with survival, regeneration and power in the world, the heart chakra is where compassion for others begins.

Graphic: Heart Chakra Pivot

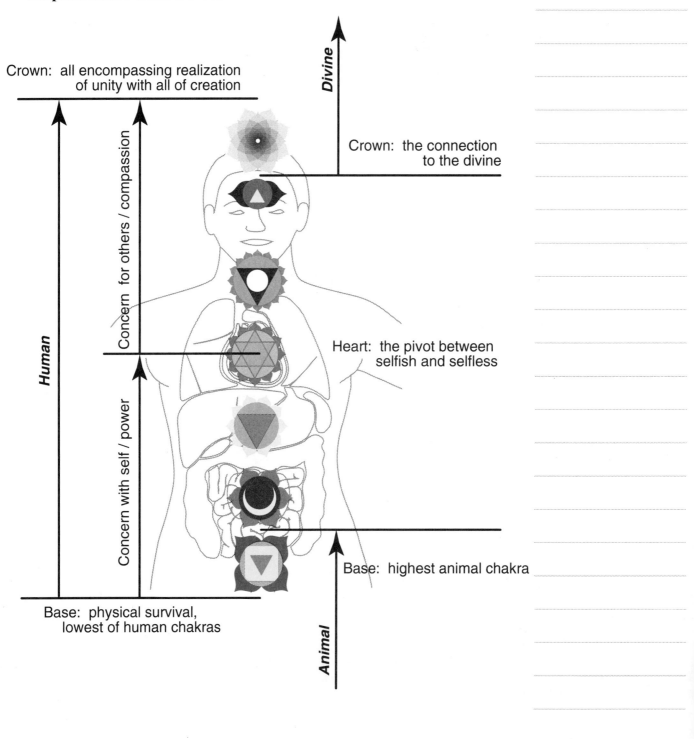

Crown: all encompassing realization of unity with all of creation

Concern for others / compassion

Human

Concern with self / power

Base: physical survival, lowest of human chakras

Divine

Crown: the connection to the divine

Heart: the pivot between selfish and selfless

Base: highest animal chakra

Animal

Chakra #5, Throat

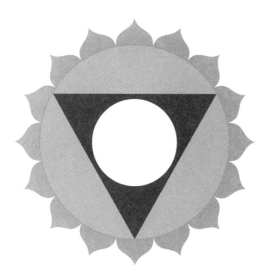

This is the chakra located in the throat and is thus related to communication and self-expression through creativity. Here we experience the world symbolically through vibration, such as the vibration of sound representing language.

This is the chakra that has the power of speech and manifestation through words. Balance here is expressed by clarity in speech, thought and action.

Chakra #6, Third Eye

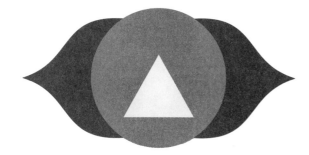

This chakra is known as the brow chakra or third eye center, its associated element is light. It is related to the act of seeing, both physically and intuitively and allows for self-reflection. As such it opens our mind and our understanding.

When healthy it allows us to see clearly, in effect, letting us "see the big picture."

Ajna is the site of intuitive wisdom.

Chakra #7, Crown

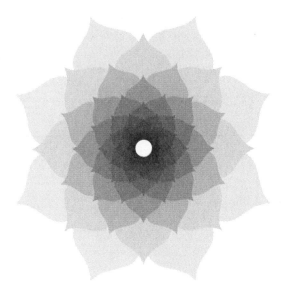

This is the crown chakra that relates to consciousness as pure awareness. It is our connection to the greater world and beyond. It transcends time and space. It is all knowing without thought, oriented to self-knowledge.

When developed, this chakra brings us knowledge, wisdom, understanding, spiritual connection, and bliss.

Name	Root / Base	Sacral / Naval	Solar Plexus	Heart	Throat	Brow / Third Eye	Crown
#	1	2	3	4	5	6	7
Sanskrit Name	Muladhara (root/support)	Svadhisthana (sweetness)	Manipura (lustrous jewl)	Anahata (unstruck)	Visshudha (purification)	Ajna (to perceive)	Sahasrara (thousandfold)
Location	Base of spine	AbdomenGenitals lower back, hips	Solar Plexus	Heart "area"	Throat	Third Eye	Top of Head
Color	red	orange	yellow	green	blue	indigo	violet
Orientation to self	Self-preservation to be here,	Self-gratification	Self-definition	Self-acceptance	Self-expression	Self-reflection	Self-knowledge
Rights	to have	to feel, to want	to act	to love and be loved	to speak and be heard	to see	to know
Central Issue	Survival, grounding	Sexuality, emotions, desire	Power, will	Love, relationships	Communication	Intuition, imagination	Awareness
Qualities	Stability, grounding, physical health, prosperity, trust	Fluidity, pleasure, healthy sexuality, feeling	Vitality, spontaneity, strength of will, purpose, self-esteem	Balance, compassion, self-acceptance, good relationships	Clear communication, creativity, resonance	Psychic perception accurate interpretation, imagination, clear seeing	Wisdom, knowledge, consciousness
Element	Earth	Water	Fire	Air	Sound	Light	Information
Identity	Physical	Emotional	Ego	Social	Creative	Archetypal	Universal
Demon	Fear	Guilt	Shame	Grief	Lies	Illusion	Attachment
Excessive Attributes	Heaviness, Sluggish monotony, obesity, hoarding, materialism, greed	Overly emotional, poor boundaries, sex addiction, obsessive attachments	Dominating, blaming, aggressive, scattered, constantly active	Codependency, poor boundaries, possessive, jealous	Excessive talking, inability to listen, over-extended, stuttering	Headaches nightmares, delusions, difficulty concentrating	Overly intellectual, spiritual addiction, confusion, dissociation
Deficient Attributes	Frequent fear, lack of discipline, restless, underweight, spacey	Frigidity, impotence, rigidity, emotional numbness, fear of pleasure	Weak will, poor self esteem, passive, sluggish, fearful	Shy, lonely, isolated, lack of empathy, bitter, critical	Fear of speaking, poor rhythm	Poor memory, poor vision, can't see patterns, denial	Learning difficulties, spiritual apathy, skepticism, limited beliefs, materialism
Incense	cedar	orris root, gardenia	carnation	lavender, jasmine	frankincense, benzoin	mugwort, star anise	lotus, gotu kola
Gems	Lodestone, ruby, garnet, hematite smoky quartz, obsidian, onyx, jet, bloodstone, red jasper	carnelian, coral, agate, jacinth	amber, topaz, citrine quartz, tiger eye,	emerald, tourmaline, rose quartz, emerald,	turquoise, lapis lazuli, chrysocolla, green aventurine	lapis, quartz, sodalite, blue sapphire,	amethyst, diamond, white chalcedony, moss agate, desert rose, white opal, moonstone
Deities	Gaia, Auriel	Diana, Neptune, Pan, Gabriel	Amon-Ra, Brigit, Athene, Michael	Aphrodite, Frejya, Christ,	Mercury Apollo	Tara, Isis, Themis	Zeus, Nut, Inanna

Graphic: The Chakras

The Chakras

7. Crown, Sahasrana
Element: none *Planet:* none
Quality: Self transcendence, connection to universe
Sense: perception of time, infinity *Gland:* none/Pineal
Stones: Diamond, Fluorite, Amethyst
Oil: Frankinsense, Spikenard, Myrth

Note: The elements associated with the chakras are NOT the same as the five elements in TCM theory.

6. Third Eye, Ajna
Element: Ether (Light) *Planet:* Saturn
Quality: Seat of consciousness, enlightenment
Sense: Insight *Gland:* Pituitary, Pineal
Stones: Lapis Lazuli, Saphire, Azurite
Oil: Sandalwood, Frankinsense,
Clary Sage, Cardamon, Lemon

5. Throat, Vishuddha
Element: Ether *Planet:* Jupiter
Quality: Communication, self expression, creativity
Sense: Hearing *Gland:* Thyroid, parathyroid
Stones: Turquoise, Celestite, Aquamarine
Oil: Rosemary, Sage, Spike Lavender,
Black Spruce, Patchouli

4. Heart, Anahata
Element: Air *Planet:* Venus
Quality: Love, conectedness, balance
Sense: Touch *Gland:* Thymus
Stones: Emerald, Jade, Rose Quarz
Oil: Rose, Palmarosa, Neroli,
Lavender, Bergamot

3. Solar Plexus, Manipura
Element: Fire *Planet:* Sun
Quality: Aspiration, Ego
Sense: Vision *Gland:* Pancreas
Stones: Citrine, Tiger Eye, Gold
Oil: Black Pepper, Cardamon, Sweet
Orange, Vetiver

2. Sacral, Naval, Svadisthana
Element: Water *Planet:* Mercury
Quality: Flow, sexuality, family and friends
Sense: Taste *Gland:* Testes, Ovaries
Stones: Coral, Amber, Citrine, Gold Topaz
Oil: Jasmine, Neroli, Patchouli, Geranium

1. Base, Root, Muladhara
Element: Earth *Planet:* Mars
Quality: Grounding, physical stamina
Sense: Smell *Gland:* Adrenals
Stones: Ruby, Hematite, Smoky Quarz
Oil: Cedar, Sandalwood, Vetiver, Cypress, Juniper

Note: Acording to some sources the hands and feet are the sites of secondary chakras, minor chakras are also located at the nape of the neck, along the spine and in the genital area

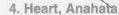

Notes

Addendum
TCM Booklist

Chinese Medicinal Wines and Elixirs, Bob Flaws, Blue Poppy Press, 1994

Tao; the Subtle Universal Law and the Integral Way of Life, Hau-Ching Ni, Sevenstar Communications, 1979, 1983

Tao of Physics, Fritjof Capra, Shambhala, 1975

The Tao of Sex, Howard S. Levy and Akira Ishihara, Harper and Row, 1968, 1989

Dragon Rises Red Bird Flies; Psychology and Chinese Medicine, Leon Hammer MD, Station Hill Press, 1990

Healing With Whole Foods; Oriental Traditions and Modern Nutrition, Paul Pitchford, North Atlantic Books, 1993

The Web That Has No Weaver, Ted Kaptchuk OMD, Contemporary Books, 1983, 2000

Acupuncture Charts, Liu Zhaoyuan Prof., China Cultural Corporation, 1975

The Art of War, Sun-Tzu, Ralph D. Sawyer, Barnes&Noble, 1994

My Sister The Moon; The Diagnosis & Treatment of Menstrual Disease by Traditional Chinese Medicine, Bob Flaws, Blue Poppy Press, 1994

The Essence of Feng Shui, Jami Lin, Hay House Inc., 1998

Feng Shui, JohnDennis Govert, Daikakuji Publications, 1993

The Feng Shui Handbook, Derek Walters, Aquarian Press, 1991

Feng Shui; A Layman's Guide to Chinese Geomancy
Feng Shui for Business
Feng Shui for the Home, Evelyn Lip, Heian International, 1990

Ayurveda Booklist

Ayurveda: The Science of Self-Healing, Usha Lad, Dr. Vasant Lad; Ayurvedic Press, Albuquerque, 1994

The Yoga of Herbs, David Frawley and Dr. Vasant lad, Lotus Press, 1986

The Book of Ayurveda; A Holistic Approach to Health and Longevity, Judith H. Morrison, Simon & Schuster Inc., 1995

The Hidden Secret of Ayurveda, Robert E. Prakruti Svoboda, The Ayurvedic Press, Albuquerque, 1994

Life Health & Longevity, Robert E. Prakruti Svoboda, Penguin Press, 1992

Your Ayurvedic Constitution, Robert E. Prakruti Svoboda, Geocom Press, 1989

Ayurvedic Healing, David Frawley, Morison Publishing, 1989

Ayurvedic Cooking for Self-Healing, Usha Lad, Dr. Vasant Lad; Ayurvedic Press, Albuquerque, 1994

Ayurveda & Aromatherapy, Dr. Light Miller ND. & Dr. Bryan Miller DC., Lotus Press, 1995

Aromatherapy Booklist

Aromatique : A Sensualist's Guide, Eva Marie Lind, Bay Soma Publishing
ISBN:1579590691, 2002

Breathing: Expanding Your Power and Energy, Michael Sky, Bear&Co., 1990

Vibrational Healing, Deborah Eidson, Frog Lmtd., 2000

Chakras; Balance your Body's Energy for Health and Harmony, Patricia Mercier, Godsfield Press, 2000

Subtle Aromatherapy, Patricia Davis, CW Daniel, 1991

Aromatherapy for Healing the Spirit, Gabriel Mojay, Henry Holt Co., 1996

The Garden of Life, Naveen Aquarian Press/Harper Collins, 1993

Colour Energy for Body and Soul, Inger Naess, 1998, www.colourenergy.com

Mandala; Luminous Symbols for Healing, Judith Cornell, Ph.D., Quest Books, 1994

The Healing Energies of Light, Roger Coghill, Gaia Books, 2000

Fragrant Heavens; The Spiritual Dimension of Fragrance &Aromatherapy, Valerie Ann Worwood, New World Library, 1999

TCM Schools

This list is by no means complete and inclusion is not endorsement check them out if you want to know more.

Academy of Chinese Culture and Health Sciences
1601 Clay Street
Oakland, CA 94612

Academy of Oriental Medicine at Austin
2700 West Anderson Lane, Suite 117
Austin, TX 78757

American College of Acupuncture
1021 Park Avenue
New York, NY 10028

American College of Traditional Chinese Medicine
455 Arkansas Street
San Francisco, CA 94107

Arizona School of Acupuncture and Oriental Medicine
4646 East Fort Lowell Rd., #105
Tucson, AZ 85712

Bastyr University
14500 Juanita Drive NE
Bothell, WA 98011

China International Medical University
822 S. Robertson Blvd., Ste. 300-303
Los Angeles, CA 90035

Colorado School of Traditional Chinese Medicine
1441 York Street, Suite 202
Denver, CO 80206

Emperor's College of Traditional Oriental Medicine
1807-B Wilshire Blvd.
Santa Monica, CA 90403

Five Branches Institute:
College of Traditional Chinese Medicine
200 7th Ave.
Santa Cruz, CA 95062

Institute of Clinical Acupuncture and Oriental Medicine
1270 Queen Emma Street #107
Honolulu, HI 96813

International Institute of Chinese Medicine
P.O. Box 29988
Santa Fe, NM 87592-9988

Life Circles School of Healing Arts
965 East 28th Street
Ogden, UT 84403

Meiji College of Oriental Medicine
2550 Shattuck Ave.
Berkeley, CA 94704

National College of Naturopathic Medicine
049 SW Porter
Portland, OR 97201

NIAOM
701 N 34th. St, Ste. 300
Seattle, WA 98103

Northwest Institute of Acupuncture
and Oriental Medicine
701 N. 34th St. #300
Seattle, WA 98103

Oregon College of Oriental Medicine
10525 SE Cherry Blossom Dr.
Portland, OR 97216

Pacific College of Oriental Medicine
7445 Mission Valley Rd. Suites 103-106
San Diego, CA 92108

Samra University of Oriental Medicine
3000 S. Robertson Blvd., 4th Floor
Los Angeles, CA 90034

Santa Barbara College of Oriental Medicine
1919 State Street, Suite 204
Santa Barbara, CA 93101

Seattle Institute of Oriental Medicine
916 NE 65th, Suite B
Seattle, WA 98115

South Baylo University
1126 N. Brookhurst Street
Anaheim, CA 92801

Tai Hsuan Foundation, Acupuncture
and Herbal Medicine College
2600 S. King Street #206
Honolulu, HI 96726

Western States Chiropractic College
2900 NE 132nd Avenue
Portland, OR 97230

Yo San University of Traditional Chinese Medicine
13315 West Washington Blvd. Ste. 200
Los Angeles, CA 90066

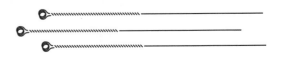

Quiz 1

1. ___ Chinese Medicine is based on the concept of:
   a) Flow of Qi
   b) Flow of Karma
   c) Balance of Fluids
   d) Balance of Fire, Water, Earth, Air

2. ___ Yin and Yang are:
   a) Interdependent
   b) Mutually controlling
   c) Philosophical constructs
   d) all of the above

3. ___ Match Yin and Yang to the following pairs:

solid _____   liquid _____
hot _____   cold _____
day _____   night _____
female _____   male _____
steam _____   liquid _____
heaven _____   earth _____

4. ___ The generating order of the Five Elements is:
   a) Fire, Water, Earth, Wood, Metal
   b) Earth, Wind, and Fire, Sound, Good
   c) Water, Wood, Fire, Earth, Metal
   d) Water, Earth, Wood, Fire, Metal

5. ___ Acupuncture needles stimulate:
   a) Capillary beds
   b) Immune system
   c) Nerves
   d) Yin/Yang
   e) Qi

6. ___ The Element that corresponds to the center of a compass is:
   a) Fire
   b) Water
   c) Earth
   d) Wood

7. ___ Winter is the domain of what Element?
   a) Fire
   b) Water
   c) Earth
   d) Wood

Quiz 2

1. ____ According to Chinese Medicine, applying pressure or stimulating points along meridians will increase the flow of:
   a) blood
   b) prana
   c) lymph
   d) Qi

2. ____ Qi is generated by:
   a) food and water in the stomach
   b) absorption of cosmic radiation (Ether)
   c) air and food in the chest
   d) air and will in the mind

3. ____ Match Yin and Yang to the following pairs:

anterior of body _____   posterior of body _____
contracting _____   expanding _____
descending _____   ascending _____
active _____   passive _____
light _____   dark _____
order _____   chaos _____

4. ____ The controlling order of the Five Elements is:
   a) Fire, Water, Earth, Wood, Metal
   b) Fire, Metal, Wood, Earth, Water
   c) Water, Wood, Fire, Earth, Metal
   d) Water, Earth, Wood, Fire, Metal

5. ____ Which of the following organs is Yang Earth:
   a) Spleen
   b) Stomach
   c) Kidney
   d) Heart
   e) Lung

6. ____ The organ that is associated with the skin is:
   a) Lung
   b) Liver
   c) Large Intestine
   d) Small Intestine

7. ____ How many Channel Organs are there in Chinese Medicine?
   a) 8
   b) 10
   c) 12
   d) 14

Quiz 3

1. ___ In what vessel is Yin located in the body:
    a) Governing vessel (Du)
    b) Life vessel
    c) Conception vessel (Ren)
    d) Kidney channel

2. ___ What channel runs parallel to the spine:
    a) Conception vessel (Du)
    b) Urinary Bladder channel
    c) Kidney channel
    d) Stomach channel

3. ___ Match Fire, Earth, Metal, Water, Wood to the following qualities:

summer _____	sour	_____
red _____	controls sweat	_____
center _____	bones	_____
sadness _____	spring	_____
fear _____	joy	_____
shouting _____	dryness	_____

4. ___ What channel starts at the medial border of the nail of the big toe?
    a) Spleen
    b) Stomach
    c) Kidney
    d) Heart
    e) Lung

5. ___ What channel is responsible for the smooth flow of emotions?
    a) Liver
    b) Stomach
    c) Kidney
    d) Heart
    e) Lung

6. ___ Pain can be the result of:
    a) stagnation of Qi
    b) stagnation of Blood
    c) Hypochondria
    d) all of the above

7. ___ What channel runs across the nipples and over the abdomen ?
    a) Spleen
    b) Stomach
    c) Small Intestine
    d) Heart

Quiz 4

1. Draw and label the Kidney channel:
2. Draw and label the Urinary Bladder channel:
3. Mark and label the beginning of the Lung channel:

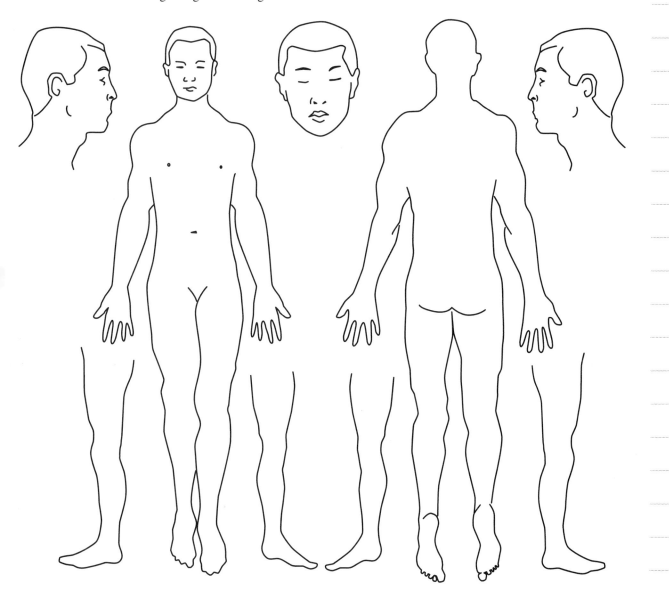

4. ___ What channel is afflicted when the patient presents with fear:
   a) Conception vessel (Du)
   b) Urinary Bladder channel
   c) Kidney channel
   d) Stomach channel

5. ___ Addiction would likely be treated with:
   a) Jail
   b) Ear acupuncture
   c) Foot reflexology
   d) Iridology

4. ___ What channel starts in the axilla?
     a) Spleen
     b) Stomach
     c) Kidney
     d) Heart
     e) Lung

True or false?

5.   You have to believe in acupuncture in order for it to work
          T   F

6.   Chinese Medicine can not help with emotional disorders
          T   F

7.   Acupuncture works best with Chinese Medical Diagnosis
          T   F

8.   Lifestyle is negligible on the course of an infection
          T   F

9.   Only top grade medicinal herbs have medicinal functions
          T   F

10.   Acupuncture can make me stop smoking
          T   F

11.   Acupuncture will leave scars
          T   F

12.   There is good pain there is bad pain
          T   F

13.   Chinese Medicine can't treat modern diseases because its too old
          T   F

14. ___ Chinese herbal weight loss pills are:
     a) safe because they are made of herbs
     b) only to be taken after consultation with nutritionist
     c) only to be taken after consultation with naturopath
     d) only to be taken after consultation with Chinese Medicinal Herbalist
     e) only to be taken after consultation with a western medical doctor

15. ___ The tongue will reflect:
     a) the condition of the Qi in the body
     b) the condition of the internal organs
     c) the presence of pain
     d) all of the above

16. ___ The best way to support weight loss is:
     a) watch TV and wait for QVC to sell exercise equipment
     b) use triple dose secret Hollywood Superstar Fat burn Metabolizer
     c) eat only non-fat foods
     d) join the eat-all-you-want-and-get-still-get-slim herbal diet
     e) exercise

What would you like to know about oriental medicine? Suggestions?
Comments?

Thanks to Michael Matthes for technical help, my wife Anna for keeping me on track and to my many students for their questions and feedback.